Integrating UK and European Social Policy
The Complexity of Europeanisation

Robert Geyer

and

Andrew Mackintosh

with

Kai Lehmann

Foreword by

Ian Bache

Radcliffe Publishing
Oxford ● Seattle

Radcliffe Publishing Ltd
18 Marcham Road
Abingdon
Oxon OX14 1AA
United Kingdom

www.radcliffe-oxford.com
Electronic catalogue and worldwide online ordering facility.

British Library Cataloguing in Publication Data

A catalogue record for this book is available from the British Library

ISBN-10: 1 85775 764 5

Typeset by Action Publishing Technology Ltd, Gloucester
Printed and bound by TJ International Ltd, Padstow, Cornwall

Contents

Foreword

Interdisciplinarity is widely preached and yet rarely practised. But perhaps this should not be too surprising. While its advantages are ever clearer in that many issues are increasingly complex and rarely understood from a single disciplinary position, academic institutions and debates remain generally organised around traditional disciplinary concerns. Overcoming these constraints generally requires challenging both established ideas and interests. This book embraces this challenge. In doing so, the authors bring together the academic themes of complexity and Europeanisation, both of which are ripe for interdisciplinary engagement.

Complexity theory seeks to build a bridge between rationalist and post-modern approaches to enquiry. It demands, as the authors put it, 'a broad and open-minded approach to epistemological positions and methodological strategies without universalising particular positions or strategies'. Phenomena may be orderly or disorderly: the key is to recognise the difference between the two and acknowledge the limits to prediction in relation to the latter. The theory emerged from the natural sciences before spilling over into the social sciences and now provides a new departure in the study of the European Union (EU).

From a complexity perspective, the EU has both elements of orderliness and disorderliness. It has a relatively stable institutional framework, yet there are divergent patterns of activity and outcome. It allows for a degree of coherence and divergence at the same time and, as the authors suggest, 'the very messiness of the EU is one of its major hidden strengths'. Nowhere is this paradox of coherence and divergence more apparent than in the relations between the EU and its member states and, more specifically, in the domestic effects of EU membership: the notion of Europeanisation.

Europeanisation is itself a relatively new field of enquiry. While the term has existed for a while, and has been used to describe a wide range of phenomenon, conceptual refinement has been relatively recent and its empirical focus has settled on domestic change. It draws heavily on the insights of new institution-alism and multi-level governance, both of which acknowledge complexity, and highlights both convergent and divergent outcomes from the complex interplay of EU and domestic forces and processes.

In this context, the prospects for complexity theory in relation to study of European integration generally and Europeanisation specifically appear promising. The EU represents a novel form of organisation that is ripe for interdisciplinary understanding of the complex interrelationship of cultural, economic, legal, political and social aspects. It is neither exclusively national, nor domestic; rational, nor post-modern; orderly, nor disorderly.

In *Integrating UK and European Social Policy: the Complexity of Europeanisation*, the authors seek to carry this research agenda forward in a practical manner. The framework of complexity theory is combined with a detailed study of the British–EU social policy relationship. The book is a bold attempt to combine theoretical innovation with detailed policy analysis. Whether the authors manage this delicate balancing act or not only the reader can decide. However, for attempting this task, and for embracing the challenge of interdisciplinary enquiry, this book makes a contribution to the study of Europeanisation that undoubtedly deserves to be read.

Ian Bache
Department of Politics, University of Sheffield
Convenor of the ESRC seminar series and UACES study group on
the Europeanisation of British politics and policymaking
www.shef.ac.uk/ebpp/
June 2005

Preface

So quick bright things come to confusion
(Shakespeare, *A Midsummer Night's Dream*)

This book began as the second part of a research project into the fate of the European social model and welfare state. The roots of this project can be found in the fears for that model and welfare state that grew up in the 1980s and 1990s around the growing forces of Europeanisation and globalisation. Under such conditions, could the EU save Social Europe or was it actively undermining it? An obvious first step was to see just what the European Union (EU) was doing in the field of social policy. This led to the book, *Exploring European Social Policy* (Geyer 2000c) and the conclusion that the EU social policy regime was not replacing or undermining national welfare states, but interacting with them in unique, complex and divergent ways. Clearly, the second step was to study the interaction between a member state, the UK, and the EU social regime. This could then be brought together with other national studies to create a coherent comparative picture.

After obtaining generous funding from the Nuffield Foundation to support the project, we got on with the work of conducting our elite interviews, tracing policy documents and reviewing academic sources. However, as we were proceeding smoothly down this interesting but rather conventional path, we kept running into the problem of complexity. For example, there never seemed to be a central actor or dynamic to the EU–UK social regime relationship. Most actors only knew part of the EU–UK relationship and had no idea what was going on outside their particular specialism. Moreover, despite the controlling hand of some type of managing actor, stable policy dynamics (day-to-day interactions, long-term strategies, etc) did emerge relatively smoothly. However, these were never stable enough for us to find complete causality or certain predictability. At some level, the EU–UK relationship was constantly evolving and varied depending upon which aspect one looked at. We had a growing sense of desperately attempting to take a picture of a fast-flowing river while trying to keep track of certain eddies or whorls (particularly policy areas). Yet at the same time, we had to keep in mind that there were currents underneath (larger global and European political and economic forces) that were constraining and directing these eddies and whorls. Hence, from the very beginning we were confronted with a sense of failure at not being able to fully capture the picture of the river in all of its detail, nor to grasp the essence of the relationship between the deeper flows and surface manifestations.

This sense of frustration led us in two directions. First, we decided to reduce the number of social policy arenas that we would examine. Our original plans included exploring between 8–10 social policy areas, a respectable goal but clearly beyond the boundaries of what we wanted to achieve. Second, we began looking for a new way to understand the complexity that we were seeing. A pathway emerged in the unlikely shape of one of our colleagues at the

University of Liverpool, Samir Rihani. Though in the School of Politics and Communications Studies, Samir had an engineering education and broad experience in local government and business. It was Samir who first pushed the idea of complexity theory into our heads (though we did our best to resist) and gave us the courage to try to link it into our particular field of politics. After that there was no going back, and the result lies in front of you. Robert Geyer became so involved in complexity that he and Samir went on to establish the University of Liverpool Complexity Network and Centre for Complexity Research (www.liv.ac.uk/ccr). If the arguments in the book intrigue you, we encourage you to take a look at the website.

Please note, sections of Chapter 2 and 3 are drawn from Robert Geyer's articles 'European integration, the problem of complexity and the revision of theory' (Geyer 2003a); 'Beyond the Third Way: the science of complexity and politics of choice' (Geyer 2003b); 'The end of globalisation and Europeanisation, rise of complexity and future of Scandinavian exceptionalism' (Geyer 2003c). The section on EU social policy in Chapter 1 is drawn from Robert Geyer's book *Exploring European Social Policy* (Geyer 2000c) and the book chapter 'Britain in the European Union' in Ellison and Pierson (2003) *New Developments in British Social Policy*. Robert Geyer and Andrew Macintosh were the primary authors. Kai Lehmann was responsible for Chapter 1.

As is the norm for the end of prefaces we have a number of institutions and people to thank. Financial support from the University of Liverpool Research Development Fund and a grant from the Nuffield Foundation were essential for giving us the time to work and ability to perform our London- and Brussels-based interviews. We would like to thank the more than 120 interviewees who gave us their time and opinions. Almost all were friendly and supportive of our research. We have intellectual debts that are too numerous to mention. However, of special note is the friendship and support of Dr Samir Rihani. Lastly, we would like to thank our families and friends for helping us along our intellectual journey. We hope the reader finds it interesting and as useful as we did.

Robert Geyer
Andrew Mackintosh
Kai Lehmann
June 2005

About the authors

Dr Robert Geyer (PhD University of Wisconsin-Madison) has been working on issues of international political economy, European integration and social policy for past 15 years at the University of Wisconsin, Marquette University and University of Liverpool. He has published two single-authored books and over 25 articles and book chapters in these areas. In the past five years he has been captivated by the ability of complexity to reshape the fundamental understanding of these fields and create new interdisciplinary linkages between the social and natural sciences. This led him to found, in 2002, and currently direct the Centre for Complexity Research at the University of Liverpool (www.liv.ac.uk/ccr).

Andrew Mackintosh (MPhil University of Liverpool) focuses on the policy dynamics of the European Union and their implications for British policy development. He has been exploring the implications of complexity to this field for the past four years and has been a member of the Centre for Complexity Research since its founding. He is currently a researcher linked to the Centre for Complexity Research and works on employment policy.

Kai Lehmann (PhD candidate, University of Liverpool) is an expert in European integration, international relations and complexity. His current work uses complexity theory to understand the role of crises and 'shock events' in the formation of US, UK and German foreign and national policy. He has worked in the UK Cabinet Office and is a researcher and postgraduate coordinator at the Centre for Complexity Research.

Abbreviations

ACAS	Advisory Conciliation and Arbitration Service
ARD	Acquired Rights Directive
BECTU	Broadcasting, Entertainment, Cinematograph and Theatre Union
BEPGs	Broad Economic Policy Guidelines
CAC	Central Arbitration Committee
CAP	Common Agricultural Policy
CBI	Confederation of British Industry
CEEP	Centre Européen des enterprises à participation publique et des enterprises d'intérêt économique general
CRD	Collective Redundancies Directive
CTC	Children's Tax Credit
DfEE	Department for Education and Employment
DfES	Department for Education and Skills
DH	Department of Health
DPTC	Disabled Person's Tax Credit
DSS	Department of Social Security
DTI	Department of Trade and Industry
DWP	Department for Work and Pensions
EAP	Employment Action Plan
EAT	Employment Appeal Tribunal
ECB	European Central Bank
ECJ	European Court of Justice
ECOFIN	Economic and Finance Council
ECS	European Company Statute
ECSC	European Coal and Steel Community
ECU	European Currency Unit
EDP	Excessive Deficit Procedure
EEA	European Economic Area
EEC	European Economic Community
EEP	European Employment Pact
EES	European Employment Strategy
EI	European integration
EIRO	European Industrial Relations Observatory
EIRR	European Industrial Relations Review
EIS	European Information Service
EMAC	Economic and Monetary Affairs Committee
EMU	European Monetary Union
EOC	Equal Opportunities Commission
EPA	Equal Pay Act
EPD	Equal Pay Directive
ERDF	European Regional Development Fund
ERM	Exchange Rate Mechanism
ESF	European Social Fund

ETD	Equal Treatment Directive
ETUC	European Trade Union Confederation
EU	European Union
EWC	European Works Council
EWCB	European Works Councils Bulletin
EWCD	European Works Councils Directive
EWL	European Women's Lobby
FCO	Foreign and Commonwealth Office
GDP	Gross domestic product
HAD	Horizontal Amending Directive
ICD	Information and Consultation Directive
ICT	Information computer technology
IGC	Intergovernmental conference
IMF	International Monetary Fund
IR	International relations
JER	Joint employment record
JSA	Jobseekers' Allowance
LPC	Low Pay Commission
MA	Maternity Allowance
MEP	Member of the European Parliament
MLG	Multilevel Governance
MP	Member of Parliament
MPC	Monetary Policy Committee
NAPs	National action plans
ND25plus	New Deal for the over 25s
NDYP	New Deal for Young People
NGOs	Non-governmental organisations
NHS	National Health Service
NICs	National Insurance Contributions
NOW	New Opportunities for Women
ODPM	Office of the Deputy Prime Minister
OMC	Open method of coordination
PAET	Policy Appraisal for Equal Treatment
PSNB	Public sector net borrowing
PT	Policy transfer
QMV	Qualified majority voting
RDA	Regional development agency
SAP	Social Action Programme
SDA	Sex Discrimination Act
SE	Societas Europaea
SEA	Single European Act
SGP	Stability and Growth Pact
SMEs	Small and medium sized enterprises
SMP	Statutory Maternity Pay
SNB	Special negotiating body
SPP	Statutory Paternity Pay
TEU	Treaty of European Union
TUC	Trades Union Congress
TUPE	Transfer of Undertakings (Protection of Employment) Regulation

UN	United Nations
UNICE	Union des Industries de la Communauté Européene
VAT	Value Added Tax
WEU	Women and Equality Unit
WFTC	Working Families' Tax Credit
WIRS	Workplace Industrial Relations Survey
WTD	Working Time Directive
WTR	Working Time Regulations
WWII	World War II

Introduction

In the late 1980s and early 1990s, as European integration rapidly accelerated, debates raged over the impact of the European Union (EU) on member state policy arenas. Regarding member state welfare state regimes, a common fear on the left was that EU social policy and Europeanisation would inevitably encourage member state welfare state regimes to converge around a European norm, raising fears of a destructive race to the bottom (Stewart 1984; Cerny 1990; Scharpf 1991; Moses 1994; Teeple 1995). On the other hand, the right feared that new EU social policies would wreck European competitiveness and block successful national level welfare state liberalisation plans. Margaret Thatcher's famous Bruges speech on rolling back the state encapsulated this position. However, as the 1990s progressed, both fears were found to be unsubstantiated. Many welfare states successfully resisted significant international constraints and anti-welfarist political movements, disproving the convergence hypothesis (Boyer and Drache 1996; Hirst and Thompson 1996; Swank 1998). Likewise, as EU social policy evolved in the 1990s and moved away from its earlier emphasis on harmonisation and towards a much more cooperative and consensual direction, the threat of an oppressive EU welfare state became increasingly unjustifiable. Between these two poles, others (Geyer 1997, 2000a; Hine and Kassim 1998; Rhodes and Meny 1998; Sykes and Alcock 1998) attempted to go beyond these earlier interpretations and argue that the EU's impact was much more variable, complex and uncertain. In essence, similar to the latest debates surrounding the development and impact of globalisation, Europeanisation can no longer be seen as a coherent hegemonic force that will have a unifying effect on political arenas and policy areas. Given this variable and interrelated relationship, the central question becomes how EU social policy *interacts* with UK social policy, rather than how it *impacts* upon it.

This conclusion mirrors a general 'complexity' (Kiel and Elliot 1997; Byrne 1998; Cilliers 1998; Rihani 2002) shift in European integration and welfare state theory. In essence, this has led away from a strong belief in the orderly/rational nature of society, the ability of the state to pursue and obtain clear objects, and the ability of the researcher to fully capture and understand societal relationships in a reductionist manner. For example, the traditional debate within European integration theory was between intergovernmentalists, espousing the dominance of the EU member states in the development and implementation of EU policy, and neo-functionalists, promoting the importance of European level over national dynamics. During the 1990s, theorists using a 'multilevel governance' approach (Marks *et al.* 1996a; Sandholtz 1996; Hooghe and Marks 2001; Rosamond 2000) began to argue that EU development was becoming much more multilevel and interactive. National demands and positions were being interwoven with the EU level to create 'a set of over-arching, multi-level policy networks ... [where] the structure of political control is variable, not constant, across policy areas' (Rosamond 2000: 110).

Similarly, this book argues that the EU has created a new level of supra-national policy activity that alters the political arenas and policy outcomes of national and subnational systems. However, due to the complexity and relative weakness of the EU (particularly in the arena of social policy), the outcome of this interaction is both unclear and closely related to the dynamics of the national and subnational actors. Consequently, the EU is not a hegemonic actor that imposes a given structure on national systems, but an arena where national and subnational actors may be able to alter or restructure their own national and subnational arenas and strategies. Under this system, policy outcomes remain predominately national. However, the development of the EU level allows for new combinations and outcomes to occur within the fundamentally nationally based systems.

In social policy theory, traditional debates centred around a left–right axis (Glennerster 2000). On the left (particularly within the social democratic tradition), social policy and the welfare state represented a central strategy for addressing the imbalances of the market and the possibility of 'decommodifying' society (Esping-Andersen 1985). Meanwhile, the right saw social policy as an inefficient, burdensome intrusion on the market that was contrary to economic efficiency and fundamental freedoms and created a culture of dependency. Again, during the 1990s a number of theorists began to go beyond the dualistic nature of this debate. A key example was the work of Anthony Giddens (1994, 1998, 2000). In brief, Giddens argued that the restructuring of the welfare state was being defined by four major developments: the intensification of globalisation, an emerging 'post-traditional social order' (breaking out of former clear social roles), the growth of 'social reflexivity' (the growth of new flexible social identities) and 'manufactured uncertainty/risk' (the growth of uncertainty/risks related to human rather than natural intervention). To respond to these developments, advanced industrial states needed to promote 'the social investment state, operating in the context of a positive welfare society' (Giddens 1998: 117). The social investment state would focus welfare provisions on the development of social resources (training, education, social inclusion, etc), while the positive welfare society would promote these strategies through a flexible combination of state provision and alliances with civil and private organisations. Fundamentally, the overall strategy is based on making social policy and the welfare state more flexible in order to respond to the more variable and complex needs of society, and had a significant British and international impact (Department of Social Security (DSS) 1998, 1999).

Interestingly, during the 1990s the EU began to develop a similar 'flexible and adaptive' approach to its social policy. As summarised in Geyer (2000b) and Hantrais (2002), due to changes in the European Commission and continued member state resistance to significant social policy legislation, the Commission began to move away from a social policy strategy of harmonisation and towards a more consensual and cooperative approach which emphasised subsidiarity, flexible adaptation and 'best practice'. As a major Commission consultation document stated in 1993:

> *The aim is not the harmonisation of national systems, but a framework for efforts to strengthen social protection systems and enable Community legislation on social policy to fit into a dynamic framework based on common objectives* (European Commission 1993b: 44).

This flexible and learning-based approach to social policy development is very similar to Giddens' approach and the British Labour Government's 'third way' programme (Powell 1999). Consequently, the interaction of EU and UK social policy regimes raises a number of interesting questions. Most importantly, if, how and in what ways will the interaction affect the implementation of the 'positive welfare state' in Britain?

Next steps

Due to the pluralistic, multilevel, interactive and evolving nature of the EU–UK social policy relationship, one must use a variety of theoretical and method-ological tools in order to understand the relationship as fully as possible. This book will use a combination of macro-level complexity theory to discuss the evolution of traditional meso-level theories of Europeanisation and UK social policy. We will argue that these meso-level theories have become increasingly complex and receptive to the complexity of modern life in the end of the 20th century. However, they still remained mired in unproductive traditional debates over the scientific foundations of their theories and divisions between 'modernist' and 'post-modernist' positions. We believe that complexity theory allows one to go beyond the traditional linear Newtonian framework that has shaped the social sciences throughout much of the 19th and 20th centuries, and in doing so build a bridge between 'modernist' and 'post-modernist' interpreta-tions of both Europeanisation and UK social policy.

What is complexity theory and why does it help one go beyond the current debates in European integration and social policy theory? Complexity theory, developed in the natural sciences in the mid-20th century and spilling over into the social sciences from the 1980s onwards, is a new and exciting paradigmatic approach to the social sciences. As will be discussed more thoroughly in Chapter 3, complexity theory breaks with the rationalist, positivist and reductionist approaches of traditional linear social science by asserting that the natural and human worlds are composed of constantly interacting orderly and disorderly phenomena. Consequently, there are significant limits to knowledge and the ability of humans to 'order' their surroundings and lives. Fundamentally, complexity theory argues that adaptation, transformation, evolution and learn-ing are normal and healthy human processes. Order, end states, and clear linear development are impossible and dangerous for biological entities and in partic-ular humans to pursue. This is true whether those order or end states are pure communism, markets or third ways. As will be shown, complexity theory sheds a new light on the messy, interactive, chaotic and yet very normal and healthy EU–member state relationship.

Following this theoretical discussion we will explore the validity and useful-ness of complexity to four case studies of EU–UK social policy interaction: employment policy, gender policy, labour market policy and the impact of European Monetary Union (EMU). Employment, gender and labour market policy were chosen for obvious reasons. They are key social policy areas, the EU has had a lengthy involvement in each of these areas and there is a clear histor-ical and institutional legacy of EU–UK policy interaction. Comparing these three case studies will give us a good idea of the variable and emergent nature of the

EU–UK social policy relationship. The impact of EMU was added in order to explore how a more fundamental economic policy area could influence the foundations of UK social policy. This case study is necessarily more speculative. However, since EMU could have a major impact on the UK economy and governmental finances, it is undoubtedly relevant to the future of the UK social policy. These case studies are based on over 120 interviews with EU and UK policy elites in Brussels and London and a wide range of primary and secondary materials.

Structure

The book is dived into two sections: context and theory, case studies and conclusions. The first section begins with a brief description of the relationship between Social Europe and the UK social policy regime. Chapter 1 'Contextualising the EU–UK social policy relationship', sets the scene for the forthcoming theoretical chapters. It begins with a brief overview of the development and state of the EU welfare state including its funding structure, policy contours and recent policy-making innovations, and compares them to the basic outline of the UK welfare state. Next, the chapter examines the general political context of the EU–UK social policy relationship through a brief review of the role of the government, courts and Parliament. It then goes on to examine the role of the political parties and explores whether or not Labour has made a difference to the EU–UK social policy relationship. Finally, the chapter reviews the role of social non-governmental organisations (NGOs) and the special case of regional policy in the larger EU–UK relationship, the position of UK political parties to EU social policy and the role those policies have played in the development of the parties.

Chapter 2, 'European integration, UK social policy and the problem of complexity', introduces the reader to the problem of complexity in European integration and British social policy theory. Focusing on the particular manifestation of that problem in international relations/globalisation and European integration/Europeanisation, the chapter sketches out the growing theoretical recognition of complexity within the theoretical literature and then explores how complexity theory reinterprets European integration. Similarly, by concentrating on the work of Anthony Giddens' 'third way', the chapter then goes on to explore the growth of complexity in UK social policy theory and the limits of the third way for understanding that fundamental complexity.

Following this discussion of the problem of complexity, the subsequent chapter provides a detailed introduction to complexity theory. Chapter 3, 'What is complexity theory?' begins by delving into the history of science and tracing the emergence of the paradigm of order. Based on a Newtonian vision of a clockwork universe, nature and humanity were seen as fundamentally orderly and knowable. There were an array of challengers to this paradigm, but it reigned supreme through much of the 18th, 19th and 20th centuries, structuring both the natural and social sciences. However, with the rise of studies into chaotic phenomena and complex systems, the complexity paradigm began to emerge. After a brief review of this emergence, the chapter focuses on how it has spilled over into the social sciences before exploring some of the current debates between complexity thinkers within the social sciences. It concludes with a short discussion on the implications of complexity for the politics of order.

In Chapter 4, 'Using complexity to reinterpret the EU–UK social policy relationship', we apply complexity theory directly to the debates in European integration and social policy theory. We argue that both theoretical fields have gone through a similar process of growing recognition of complexity, and an increasingly static debate between the modernist and post-modernist wings of these debates. Using complexity to reconceptualise these debates, we argue that one can go beyond these divisions and reinterpret the EU–UK welfare state relationship, arguing that the combination of a fundamentally stable framework with uncertainty and complexity are the healthy norms of that relationship.

Chapter 5, 'The European Employment Strategy and the UK: a case of coincidental convergence', looks at the arena of employment policy and explores the fundamental convergence that occurred between the EU and UK employment strategies. Starting from very different positions in the 1970s and 1980s, EU employment strategies slowly shifted towards a more market-oriented and employment-enhancing framework that mirrored the traditional British approach. Consequently, recent EU employment initiatives under the European Employment Strategy have not caused significant problems for the Labour Government to implement. In this field, convergence has occurred not because either side bent to the will of the other, but due to a coincidental convergence of economic development.

Chapter 6, 'Europe leading the way? The EU as agenda setter in British equal opportunities policy', explores the influence of the most successful area of EU social policy, equal opportunities policy, on the relatively laggard British gender policy field. Despite a slow start in the 1970s and 1980s, EU equal opportunities policy accelerated rapidly in the 1990s with the growth of influential new actors, particularly the European Women's Lobby, development of new strategies including gender mainstreaming and benchmarking, and numerous legal successes at the EU level. These developments put clear pressure on certain areas of UK gender policy and made the EU a leader in these areas.

Chapter 7, 'Regulating the labour market: the partial Europeanisation of British labour market policy', examines the tensions between the more corporatist continental labour relations systems and the more voluntarist British system. With the growing success of the single market, pressures grew for the expansion of uniform European labour regulations. British resistance to these pressures and legislative initiatives has been vociferous. Nevertheless, in some areas (in the creation of works councils and aspects of working time and participation), the European model has made significant inroads into the British framework. However, other areas have remained completely untouched. Hence, the policy arena is best typified by an uneven type of partial Europeanisation.

Chapter 8, 'Economic and monetary union: the future of the economic foundation of the UK welfare state', explores the subtle yet fundamental impact of EMU on the economic foundations (fiscal and monetary policy) of the British welfare state. Following a review of the development of EMU and British monetary and fiscal policy, it examines the impact of the European procedures on other member states' fiscal and monetary policy and discusses the potential for

EMU to lead to a deeper political union. It concludes that despite the fears of many, the EMU and euro do not fundamentally undermine the fiscal and budgetary foundations of member state welfare structures, despite its more conservative monetary requirements. Thus, in the British case, EMU is not the welfarist threat that many anti-Europeans have made it to be.

The conclusion, 'Still a journey to an unknown destination', reviews the preceding chapters and assesses the specific and general implications of the EU's interaction with the British welfare state and social policy regime. This section will address the development and usefulness of the complexity paradigm and argue that it is only through the recognition of the complex and contingent relationship between the EU and member state regimes that one can come to terms with the actual reality of the EU–member state relationship. Furthermore, the open-ended and framework-oriented nature of the current EU approach to social policy enhances the adaptability and sustainability of the UK welfare state. The exact outcomes of this EU–UK interaction are impossible to predict. However, one can be confident that a more adaptable and flexible UK welfare state will be more able to survive and adapt to the inevitable challenges that will confront it than a more internalised and isolated one.

Overall, what is really new and challenging about this book is not its introduction to complexity theory or review of EU–UK social policy interaction, but the combination of the two to come to grips with the dynamics of the EU-UK welfare state relationship. From this perspective, the EU is not a domineering superstate and the UK is not an awkward partner. Both are caught within a fundamentally healthy, evolving and adaptive complex situation that encourages symbiotic learning, adaptation and adjustment. The exact outcome of this process is unknown, but its general structure and direction are sound and worth defending from the orderly visions of militant anti- and pro-Europeans.

Chapter 1

Conceptualising the EU–UK social policy relationship

Despite its growing impact on UK social policy legislation in general and the British welfare state in particular, the various mechanisms through which the European Union (EU) interacts with the British social policy are often poorly understood. In general, the academic literature either concentrates on the so-called 'Social Europe' or UK social policy regime, but rarely discusses the interaction between the two. To prepare for our later theoretical discussion and case studies one must focus on the mechanics of EU–UK social policy interaction by examining the structure of EU social policy, the EU–UK policy process and the role of the UK Parliament, government departments, political parties and social actors in that process.

We will show that, while there is frequent interaction between the EU and UK welfare state structures, the extent and nature of this interaction varies greatly over time and between policy areas. For example, in some aspects of labour or gender policy, where there is extensive and detailed interaction, the Parliament, departments, parties and social actors all play an active role in its development and implementation. In others, such as social security and health provision, where interaction is at best indirect, most of the major actors and departments pay little or no attention to the policy and consequently have a marginal impact on its development. Overall, what we find are generally pragmatic, adaptive and evolving mechanisms for EU–UK social policy interaction that enhance the learning of central policy actors, but only in special cases, EU regional policy, do these mechanisms have a pervasive effect on non-elite local and regional actors.

What does Social Europe look like?

Coming to grips with EU social policy is a particularly difficult task since it is so different from the typical welfare state model. Most fundamentally, it has minimal funding. Even if one includes all of the various structural funds as a very general type of social policy, the total is only about $40 billion/£24 billion annually, about one-third of the EU budget, less than 0.5% of EU gross domestic product (GDP), or about $100/£60 annually per capita. By comparison, total spending on broadly defined welfare aspects in the UK currently accounts for around 60% of general government expenditure and around 25% of UK GDP, about $7500/£4500 per capita (Cochrane *et al.* 2001: 77). The total EU social budget is about the same as half of the annual budget of the NHS.

Historically, EU social policy grew out of the political/military bargains embedded in the European Coal and Steel Community (ECSC) and European Economic Community (EEC), 20th century development of West European social policy, 'embedded liberalism' (Ruggie 1982) of West European capitalism, and the need to assuage the fears of sceptical workers and trade unions (Leibfried and Pierson 1995; Falkner 1998; Hantrais 2002). Its secondary position was clearly indicated by its weak foundations in the Treaties of Paris and Rome. These treaties emphasised the need to protect and improve living and working conditions, promote early forms of Eurocorporatism and, as stated in Article 118 of the Treaty of Rome, promote policy development in:

- employment
- labour law and working conditions
- basic and advanced vocational training
- social security
- prevention of occupational accidents and diseases
- occupational hygiene
- the right of association, and collective bargaining between employers and workers.

Article 119 stated that 'men and women should receive equal pay for equal work'. Finally, Articles 123–128 dealt with the creation and operation of the European Social Fund.

Due to the general stagnation of the EEC in the 1960s, it was not until the early 1970s that significant social policy progress was again made. The 1969 Hague Summit brought social policy back onto the agenda by arguing that it was a necessary complement to the economic integration envisioned by the first proposals for European Monetary Union (EMU). As the final communiqué of the 1972 Paris Summit stated:

> [the member states] *attached as much importance to vigorous action in the social field as to achievement of economic union* ... [and considered] *it essential to ensure the increasing involvement of labour and management in the economic and social decisions of the community* (Brewster and Teague 1989: 66).

Linked to this strategy was the 1974–1976 Social Action Programme (SAP) which laid down three broad areas for policy action: the 'attainment of full and better employment', 'improvement of living and working conditions' and 'increased involvement of management and labour', and specified 35 proposals for action.

As it happened, just as this radical plan for the expansion of European social policy was created, European integration lapsed into another period of stagnation and uncertainty. Following the oil shocks and massive currency fluctuations of the early 1970s, the attempt to create EMU and a coordinated European response the crisis was abandoned. Moreover, the 1970s and early 1980s saw a number of membership changes and quarrels that crippled further European community developments.

In all three areas of the SAP, developments were limited not only by the international situation, but also by the internal structure and dynamics of the

EEC itself. The general strategy of policy 'harmonisation' undercut the ability of the EEC to reach any agreements on social policy issues. The institutional weakness of the European Parliament (not even directly elected until 1979) and the Economic and Social Committee meant that social actors, such as the European Trade Union Confederation (ETUC) and European socialists, were less capable of promoting social policies within the EEC. The power of the council and the demands of unanimous voting on all major social policy questions clearly limited their development. Finally, with the rise of Margaret Thatcher in Britain in 1979, all European social policy initiatives had to pass the barrier of militant free market ideology.

With the prevailing philosophy of revived free market liberalism, weakness of European social policy supporters, and militant opposition of the British Government, social policy in the 1985 White Paper and 1986 Single European Act (SEA) was kept to a minimum. Only Article 118a established qualified majority voting (QMV) procedures in the council:

> to encourage improvements, especially in the working environment, as regards the health and safety of workers.

Despite these limitations, the SEA did lay the foundation for late 1980s 'Social Dimension'. Comprised of the Social Charter (a listing of 12 areas of fundamental social rights) and subsequent SAP, the Social Dimension performed a delicate balancing act between general support for the internal market project and specific proposals for curbing the excesses of the common market. The charter was approved as a 'solemn declaration' (opposed by the UK) and the battle over social policy shifted to the particular elements of the 1989 SAP. A key commission strategy at the time was to try and use the QMV status of health and safety issues under Article 118a as a Trojan horse for a wide array of other policies. During this period, social policy made significant gains due to the efforts of the activist Delors Commission, the growth of European level interest group activity, and the final acceptance of European integration by the West European left.

Despite grand plans and substantial effort, the late 1980s and early 1990s produced rather limited results in European social policy. Most of the legislative elements of the Social Dimension were rejected, put on hold, or watered down. However, with the creation of the 1991 Maastricht Treaty and revival of EMU, Jacques Delors brought social and regional policy back onto the agenda. Regional policy was expanded and social policy was given a fresh impetus through a number of institutional changes (the expansion of EU Parliament powers, creation of QMV in new areas of social policy, promotion of the 'social dialogue' between capital and labour, and creation of a new form of social policy initiative by agreement between EU capital and EU labour) and the creation of the Social Protocol. This seemingly clear advance for EU social policy was complicated by the unique procedural device of the British 'opt-out' clause. Using this device, Britain was allowed to 'opt-out' of future qualified majority-approved social policies, which removed a major source (British opposition) of EU Council resistance to many EU social policies, but also greatly complicated both the legal foundation and implementation of EU social policies since they could not legally or financial affect the UK.

During the mid-1990s social policy progress remained slow, but support for it continued to build. The Maastricht Treaty, after various delays, was finally ratified in 1993. In 1994, three wealthy prosocial policy member states, Austria, Finland, and Sweden, voted to join the EU. Social policy non-governmental organisations (NGOs) continued to develop at the European level. Most importantly, in May 1997 the arch opponent of EU social policy, the British Conservative Party, was decisively defeated by the Labour Party which immediately promised to end the British social policy 'opt-out'.

During the debates preceding the 1997 Amsterdam Treaty revisions, social policy was completely overshadowed by concerns with EMU, integrating new East European members, and the new section in the treaty dealing with employment policy. With the defeat of the British Conservative Government in May 1997, the Social Protocol was quickly integrated into the basic text of the Amsterdam Treaty. The treaty gave a clear commitment to the EU to address a variety of forms of discrimination in Article 13. However, the treaty refrained from making substantial spending commitments to new social policy areas and dropped measures for improving the position of the elderly and disabled from Article 137 (Duff 1997: 73).

The subsequent Commission publication on social policy, *Social Action Programme 1998–2000* (European Commission 1998) reflected this consolidating approach. The document focused on just three main areas: jobs, skills and mobility; the changing world of work; and an inclusive society, and contained the usual array of social policy proposals, but framed many of them in the new light of employment policy. With the integration of the employment section into the Amsterdam Treaty and the subsequent creation of the employment policy guidelines, the Commission clearly saw an opportunity for justifying and expanding social policies through their linkage to employment creation.

The current state of EU social policy can be summarised in Table 1.1, taken from Geyer 2000b.

Current developments

Since the end of the 1990s, four main developments have dominated the European social agenda: the European Employment Strategy, the 2001–2006 European Social Agenda, the growth of new policy methods and the integration of new East European member states. The European Employment Strategy, which emerged out of the 1997 Amsterdam Treaty (and will be discussed in more detail later), was a spill-over from the success of EMU. It was an attempt by pro-employment actors and key member states to raise the profile of employment issues through the development of a coordinated employment strategy. This strategy had four main priorities: improving employability, development of entrepreneurship, encouraging adaptability and reinforcing equal opportunities, and was based on indirect cooperation and the open method of coordination as laid out in the Luxembourg Process (European Commission 2001a: 6). Subsequent council meetings clarified and promoted the strategy, particularly the Lisbon 2000 meeting.

The *Social Policy Agenda* was the first major document of the new employment and social affairs commissioner, Anna Diamantopoulou. In line with the emphasis on employment and the economic importance of social issues, it

Table 1.1

Policy area	Original base in the treaties	Selected current base in consolidated treaties	Attained QMV status under:
Free movement	EEC (Art. 3c, 7, 48–51)	Art. 3, 14, 39–42, 61–69	SEA (Art. 49, 54)
Health and safety	ECSC (Art. 3, 35) EEC (Art. 117, 118)	Art. 3, 136, 137, 140	SEA (Art. 118a)
Employment rights	No direct reference until Maastricht	Art. 137	Unanimous voting
Working conditions	ECSC (Art. 3) EEC (Art. 117, 118)	Art. 137	SEA (Art. 118a)
Worker participation	No direct reference until Maastricht	Art. 137	Maastricht Social Protocol (Art. 2)
Social dialogue	ECSC (Art. 46, 48) EEC (Art. 193–198 creating ESC)	Art. 136, 139	Maastricht Social Protocol (Art. 4)
Gender	EEC (Art. 119)	Art. 13, 137, 141	Maastricht Social Protocol (Art. 2)
Anti-poverty/ exclusion	EEC (Art. 2, 3)	Art. 136, 137	Maastricht Social Protocol (Art. 2)
Anti-discrimination against racism	No direct reference until Amsterdam	Art. 13	Unanimous voting
Public health	No direct reference until SEA (Art. 100a, 130r)	Art. 3, 152	Maastricht (Art. 129)
Elderly	No direct reference until Amsterdam	Art. 13	Unanimous voting
Disability	No direct reference until Amsterdam	Art. 13 and declaration at end of Amsterdam	Unanimous voting
Youth/training	EEC 50, 118, 125	Art. 149, 150	Maastricht (Art. 126, 127)

stressed that the 'guiding principle of the new Social Policy Agenda will be to strengthen the role of social policy as a productive factor' (European Commission 2000a: 7). It went on to outline 34 new proposals under the headings of job creation, working environment, promoting a knowledge-based economy, free movement, social protection, combating poverty and exclusion, gender equality, fundamental rights, combating discrimination, promoting quality in industrial relations and dealing with enlargement issues. The document promoted the adoption of 20 pieces of pending legislation, but did not specify any radically new proposals for particular legislation.

Equally important, both the European Employment Strategy and the Social Policy Agenda recognised and encouraged the development of two new and related means of social policy development: *mainstreaming* and the *open method of coordination*. In the European context, mainstreaming emerged out of the activities of gender activists who were attempting to surmount the limitations of EU social policy by bringing gender issues into the mainstream of general EU policy making (Geyer 2000a, 2001). As defined in 1998 by the Council of Europe, gender mainstreaming was:

> the [re-]organisation, improvement, development and evaluation of policy processes, so that a gender equality perspective is incorporated in all policies at all levels and at all stages, by the actors normally involved in policy making (Council of Europe 1998).

In a context of few new legislative developments and constrained budgets, mainstreaming offered gender activists a number of opportunities for expanding gender policy making, strengthening gender NGOs, influencing the agenda-setting process and raising awareness of gender issues. By 1998 most major EU social policy NGOs had mainstreaming strategies and in the Social Policy Agenda, the Commission stated that 'the use of mainstreaming as a tool will be strengthened and further developed' (European Commission 2000a: 15).

The Open Method of Coordination (OMC) grew out of the development of the Employment Guidelines process created at the Luxembourg Summit (de la Porte *et al.* 2001; Hodson and Maher 2001). As summarised in de la Porte *et al.* (2001), OMC in EU social policy developed:

> primarily because – against the background of the integration of monetary policy and the close coordination of macro-economic policy, along with a general commitment to promoting supply-side policies for flexibility and employability – national and EU authorities have recognized the need to work together on policies for social cohesion (de la Porte *et al.* 2001: 296).

The OMC involved a number of policy strategies, the most important of which was benchmarking (although mainstreaming is often included as an OMC strategy). Benchmarking involved a move away from strategies of harmonisation and central decision making and towards:

> a 'post-regulatory' approach to governance, in which there is a preference for procedures or general standards with wide margins for variation, rather than detailed and non-flexible (legally binding) rules (de la Porte *et al.* 2001: 302).

Both mainstreaming and OMC gave EU social policy supporters new tactics for promoting and developing EU social policy and for strengthening European social policy actors and supporters.

Finally, the forthcoming integration of new East European member states implies substantial challenges to existing resources for EU social and regional policy and to the politics behind those policies. The difficulties become obvious when compared to the 1994 membership expansion to include Sweden, Finland and Austria. These countries were small, wealthy, had strong social policy legacies and were strong EU social policy supporters. The new Eastern European applicants are much poorer, with larger populations (particularly Poland), have very uneven social policy regimes and have often complained about EU policies that would add regulatory burdens to their struggling economies.

Overall, one is still struck by the relative weakness of EU social policy. It has seen significant developments and is pursuing a number of innovative policy strategies. However, the impact of the EU in many of these new policy areas is noticeably limited, resulting in a couple of underfunded proposals and an action plan or two. Moreover, EU social policy actors have been innovative, because they were in such a weak position that they had no other choice. They had to link into health and safety policy in the late 1980s, and employment policy in the late 1990s and create new policy strategies because their own power base and traditional strategies were so limited. Finally, due to the Commission strategy of consolidation, continual economic difficulties in much of Western Europe and the integration of poorer East European member states, a substantial expansion of EU social policy in the near future seems extremely unlikely.

The EU–UK policy process

Despite the somewhat limited nature of social policy integration described above, European Union membership has had a considerable impact on the policy process in the UK. As two leading British politics experts state: 'One of the most significant changes that has occurred in terms of British policy making since 1973 has been the integration of Britain into the EU' (Richards and Smith 2002: 146). Most fundamentally, this is due to the primacy of EU law over national law. Therefore, many decisions that directly affect the British Government and the people are not made at Westminster but in Brussels. Furthermore, as Pilkington points out:

> Community legislation is not applied to the UK by any further UK legislation but is put into effect by way of statutory instruments or orders in Council made under Section 2(2) of the European Communities Act 1972 (Pilkington 2001: 111).

Thus, some laws made in Brussels are not subject to parliamentary debate within the UK, yet they have to be applied in the UK. This suggests that EU–UK interaction is primarily unidirectional and that the role of the UK Government is reduced to that of implementer, as opposed to initiator of legislation. However, this is a very simplistic view of the policy process. In reality, the direction and level of interaction varies greatly, depending on the policy area under discussion and the type of legislation proposed.

To begin with, EU legislation itself takes various forms. It can either be a

* **regulation:** having immediate effect
* **directive:** binding legislation, but with a wide scope of implementing discretion by the national government
* **decision:** primarily an administrative instrument
* **recommendation:** non-binding instrument.

Each of these instruments implies different levels of EU–UK interactions. In terms of sheer legislative volume, every year the EU produces around 12 000 legal instruments, of which approximately 4000 are regulations and 100 or so are directives (Pilkington 2001: 103). The vast majority of EU legal instruments, however, are 'non-political' and concern routine administrative matters, such as Common Agricultural Policy (CAP) price levels. These legal instruments shall not concern us here, despite the fact that even such routine matters involve considerable interactions between EU and national officials.

As far as substantive legislative instruments are concerned, the EU–UK interaction in the policy process involves a variety of European and national actors. At the EU level, the main social policy actors are the Council of Ministers, where national governments are represented as well as the European Commission and increasingly the European Parliament. The Commission and Parliament tend to be the strongest supporters of Social Europe. How much influence the Commission and Parliament have vis-à-vis the member states depends to a large extent on the decision-making procedure used in the Council of Ministers. In many social policy areas the Commission/Parliament have little or no influence on the policy process, as they are either not part of the EU's remit (as in social security benefits), or require unanimity in the Council of Ministers, as is the case with many aspects of employment legislation. In other areas, however, such as health and safety policy, that are subject to QMV, the social policy supporters in the Commission and Parliament can have a significant impact (Wise and Gibb 1993; Hantrais 2002; Kleinman 2002).

The role of the central government

Not surprisingly, due to its privileged position relative to other UK actors, within the Council of Ministers the UK Government is one of the central actors in EU–UK social policy formation. Through the Council of Ministers it is engaged in a continual cycle of EU–UK policy interaction. It is here that most of the negotiations about EU policy take place and most of the everyday policy decisions are made, either by the respective government ministers or by senior civil servants negotiating on behalf of national governments. How much influence an individual government can have on a particular policy development depends to a large extent on the procedures used to determine the policy, which vary between unanimity and QMV. When QMV is used to pass legislation, the scope for an individual government to stop a proposal is limited and uncertain bargaining is the result. In areas where unanimity is still used, individual governments can effectively stop legislation single-handedly as the British Conservative Government under Thatcher and Major did when they successfully halted the Commission's plans to extend the EU's remit into many areas of social and employment policy in the late 1980s and early 1990s. The Council of Ministers therefore is the place where most 'political games' are played out and where central governments appear to have the most amount of control.

However, despite the hopes (or fears) of some theorists, national governments are not the unified rational actors that they like to portray. Instead they are made up of competing departments that have established their own ways of interacting with the EU. In social policy, interaction between departments and the EU is widespread. The Department for Work and Pensions (DWP), the Department of Trade and Industry (DTI), the Department of Health (DH), the Department for Education and Skills (DfES) and the Office of the Deputy Prime

Minister (ODPM) all work in areas which can, in part at least, be classified as social policy and where the EU has at least some responsibility.

Interaction between central government and the EU can take many forms. There are obviously, as stated above, many ministerial meetings on all matters European. Such meetings are prepared by both British and EU civil servants so that extensive interaction occurs on that front. Furthermore, the work of individual departments is scrutinised by parliamentary select committees and these committees may well decide to look into how the department has dealt with a particular European issue. So, for instance, the Trade and Industry Select Committee could decide to investigate the impact of the EU Working Time Directive on British industry, or the Education and Skills Select Committee could look into the impact of the European Social Fund (ESF) on the skills base of the British workforce. There is therefore a patchwork of interaction between the two layers of government, both in terms of social policy and in other policy areas.

The exact pattern of interaction between the EU and government departments is very difficult to establish. For instance, the DfES deals with the EU on many issues. In some, such as the European Social Fund (ESF), the guidelines passed down by the Commission on how to implement it are quite clear, and the DfES is essentially an implementer. In others, such as the Commission's Employment Strategy, which will be discussed in Chapter 5, with its open method of coordination and benchmarking, interaction is more messy, but with central government essentially in control of the policy process (de la Porte *et al.* 2001; Hodson and Maher 2001). Until the 1990s, the UK's centralised political decision-making structure meant that interaction between the EU and the UK was clearly structured, linear and essentially only involved two actors: the central government and the respective EU institutions. Unsurprisingly, as our interviews showed, upper level civil servants were not opposed to this structure as it left the central government machinery in control of both policy development and implementation.

However, since the election of a Labour Government in 1997, UK central government control over the social policy process has been complicated by the creation of the devolved administrations in Wales and Scotland. Wales and Scotland used to have all their affairs, including interaction at EU level, administered and regulated from London. This has now changed significantly with the creation of the Welsh Assembly and Scottish Parliament. This is particularly important with regard to the EU's regional policy, from which Scotland and Wales have benefited significantly in the form of the European Regional Development Fund (ERDF) and the ESF. These funds are now administered directly by the Welsh Assembly and the Scottish Parliament, effectively introducing another level of interaction into the political process for these regions of the UK (DTI European Structural Funds website; Begg and Mayes 1993).

But even within the ranks of central government, the interaction between the European and the national level is not clear-cut. Most departments have some sort of involvement with the EU. On top of that there are two government departments with an overall coordinating role in relation to EU policy: the Foreign and Commonwealth Office (FCO) and the Cabinet Office. The FCO has its own 'Minister for Europe'. Interestingly though, in the UK the Minister for Europe is not of cabinet rank, unlike in most other European countries. The

FCO also has an entire division dealing with European matters, as it has divisions dealing with all other geographical areas of the world. The FCO also provides the core of the British diplomatic personnel in Brussels.

The Cabinet Office hosts the main coordinating committee for European issues, the 'Ministerial Committee on European Issues (EP)' with the following terms of reference:

> To determine the United Kingdom's policies on European Union issues; and to oversee the United Kingdom's relations with other member states and principal partners of the European Union (Cabinet Office website).

This, as one can see, is a wide-ranging, all encompassing remit which gives the committee considerable scope to act. The wide-ranging nature of its work is also reflected in its composition. Chaired by the Foreign Secretary, the committee also includes the other members of the Cabinet, including the Secretary of State for Work and Pensions, the Secretary of State for Trade and Industry and the Secretary of State for Education and Skills.

Clearly, even within central government, the multitude of competing actors can produce a significant amount of confusion and disputes. 'Turf battles', personal rivalries, 'gold-plating' (enhancing EU policies to further your own departmental agenda), simple mistakes and other complex and disorderly processes make the EU–UK central government relationship much less 'joined-up' than it is supposed to be.[1]

The role of the courts

For some, the European Court of Justice (ECJ) is one of the key social policy actors in the EU (Weiler 1991; Mattli and Slaughter 1995; Leibfried and Pierson 1996; Armstrong and Shaw 1998; Craig and Harlow 1998). With the precedence of EU over UK law within the specified boundaries of the treaties, both the ECJ and the British courts that interpret the ECJ rulings are in a position of significant power in relation to the interaction of EU–UK social policy. The role of the ECJ in the enforcement of regulations and directives has been a subject of considerable debate over the years (Burrows and Mair 1996; Gormley 1998). Nevertheless, there is little doubt that the ECJ has had significant influence over some areas of social policy. For example, according to Stein Kuhnle, 'manifold problems and dissimilarities in the application of the free movement of workers and their equal treatment in social security have brought about a wealth of ECJ jurisprudence'(Kuhnle 2000: 188).

Moreover, social policy was and is an area where the ECJ has been very active and has created a considerable body of case law, applicable throughout the EU. By 1995, the ECJ had made 323 decisions on social security coordination and 141 decisions on 'other' social policy under Article 117–125 EEC (Leibfried and Pierson 1996: 194). Examples of how ECJ decisions have impacted on the UK can be found as far back as 1974 when the court ruled against the British Government in the so-called van Duyn case, named after the Dutch woman who brought it. In its rulings the ECJ established that the British Government had no right to refuse a work permit for Ms van Duyn, establishing the primary principle of freedom of movement, arguing that 'Article 48 has direct effect and hence confers on individuals rights that are enforceable before the courts of the member states' (ECJ Case 41/74, van Duyn ECR359). Other early examples include the ECJ's role in establishing the principle that men in the UK should receive free prescriptions at the same age as women, and of equal treatment of EU citizens with respect to social security rules and regulations (Pilkington 2001: 148).

In many ways the ECJ has been at the forefront of interaction between the EU and the UK. It is also an instrument of complexity, as it 'interferes' with and complicates the supposedly clear lines of authority and policy demarcation between the EU and national governments. Clearly, this degree of complexity is greatly enhanced when one drops down to the local level where regional and local courts are forced to interpret the meaning and implications of EU law on particular social situations. As a result of this complexity, the UK central government, bound by ECJ decisions, is perhaps not quite as dominant in the social policy process as is often suggested.

The role of Parliament

Another good illustration of the complex interaction between national and European actors in the policy process is the role of the British Parliament. Since the UK Parliament has no right to veto the growing body of legislation approved by the EU, there has been a mounting debate amongst politicians and commentators about a possible loss of sovereignty and a 'hollowing out' of the state (Marks *et al.* 1996; Cram 1997). While this may be a matter of genuine concern to some, this is not to say that the British Parliament is not involved in the EU policy-making process. In fact, its indirect involvement is extensive, if somewhat toothless.

Both the House of Commons and House of Lords have procedures in place to scrutinise proposed EU legislation before it is approved by the relevant minister. The 'Scrutiny Reserve Resolution' was formalised and passed by the House of Commons in 1990, strengthened in 1998 and states that:

> no minister should give agreement to any legislative proposal or to any agreement under Titles V or VI which is still subject to scrutiny or awaiting consideration by the House (House of Commons April 1999).

The European Scrutiny Committee assesses each EU document for its legal and/or political importance, decides which documents are to be debated on the floor of the House, monitors UK ministers in the council and is charged with reviewing legal, procedural and institutional developments within the EU. In the House of Lords, the Committee consists of six subcommittees, including one, Subcommittee F, which deals with 'social affairs, education and home affairs'. Unsurprisingly, the workload of the committee is extensive: in 2002, well over 1200 EU documents and legal instruments were examined by the committee. Of these, 535 were deemed to be of legal and/or political importance, 86 were recommended for debate, of which 9 were debated on the floor of the House, while 33 were debated in standing committees (European Scrutiny Committee 2002).

This, by any standard, is a considerable workload and would, at first glance, suggest that the influence of the Parliament on EU policy making is considerable. However, these statistics give a distorted picture of the effectiveness of the current scrutiny system. As mentioned above, the committee, both in the Commons and the Lords, does not have the power to stop legislation being adopted. Furthermore, the secrecy of the European Council and the size of the committee's workload inhibit its effectiveness. As the committee's own website states:

> *Pre- and post-council meeting scrutiny will never be really effective until the council meets in public when legislating* ... [Moreover] *the main underlying problem continues to be EU Presidencies pressing for agreement on controversial proposals without allowing sufficient time for scrutiny by national parliaments* (European Scrutiny Committee 2002: 3–4).

In theory, the committee should have some form of veto power over EU legislation in the UK. In fact, it is only in matters such as the implementation and ratification of European treaties that Parliament has a veto power. At best, the committee has delaying, questioning and amending powers that are obviously limited by the Government majority on both of the committees and their unwillingness to counter the wishes of the Government.

So while the Parliament does have a formal structure for interacting with the EU policy-making process, this structure is not very powerful and does little to decentralise the system. It has little say in what is decided between the EU and central government and how the decisions taken are implemented. As our interviews confirmed, Members of Parliament (MPs) themselves are aware of their limited capacity to influence EU policy making and of the overwhelming burden on the scrutiny committees. Furthermore, there is little evidence that Parliament has either the power or the will to change this situation in the near future, nor is there an indication from either the Government or the EU that institutional reform is in the offing that would allow more interaction, for instance by opening up meetings of the Council of Ministers. Therefore, in the British social policy context, the EU has done little to alter the fundamental dominance of the Government and civil service over Parliament. Parliament can question, delay and amend, but only in a very limited number of cases.

The role of political parties: has New Labour made a difference?

So, if the interaction between the EU and the UK in the sphere of social policy has essentially been between the British Government and the institutional actors of the EU, despite pressure from devolution and the involvement of non-national actors in areas such as regional policy, then what has been the role of the political parties? Have they been defenders of centralised hierarchical control or promoters of a more complex decentralised political process? In particular, have New Labour and the 'third way' made a difference to this tendency?

To begin, it is worth remembering that the Conservative Party was, once upon a time, seen as the pro-European party while Labour was the anti-European one. It was Edward Heath who, as Conservative Prime Minister, took the UK into what was then the European Community. Even Margaret Thatcher played a prominent role in the 'Yes' campaign when membership of the Common Market was put to a popular referendum in 1975. Equally, it was Margaret Thatcher who, as Prime Minister, signed the Single European Act of 1986, the same act that replaced the need for unanimity in the Council of Ministers with QMV for social policies such as workplace health and safety and freedom of movement. Equally, John Major, Thatcher's successor, wanted to take Britain to 'the heart of Europe'. By contrast, the Labour Party, especially during the late 1970s and early 1980s, then under the leadership of Michael Foot, was very hostile to the EU, even promising in its 1983 election manifesto to take the UK out of the European Community (Labour Party 1983), something that no major political party has advocated since as official policy. Bearing these points in mind, it is interesting to note that by the 1990s it was the Tories who were seen to be 'anti-European'. The reasons for this are manifold but mainly political, and show that a party's attitude to Europe is often shaped primarily by domestic political circumstance.

Margaret Thatcher had been an enthusiastic supporter of the Single Market Programme, believing it to be very much in line with her own free market beliefs and convictions (George 1991). The SEA for her was primarily a vehicle by which the neo-liberal economic programme she pursued at home could be transplanted to the whole of the European Community. For her, there was no social dimension to the entire project. By the time she resigned in 1990, the desire of the Delors Commission and some member states to create such a dimension had become obvious and Thatcher herself became an ardent back-bench critic of any such proposal, taking many in her party with her. Therefore, the Conservatives split publicly on the issue. This split became ever more apparent in the run-up to the Maastricht negotiations and was on public display throughout the early 1990s. John Major, having won the 1992 election with a wafer-thin majority, had little choice but to take the views of the 'Eurosceptic' faction of his party into account in order to stave off a serious rebellion that would have cost him his premiership. With Thatcher's views and economic reforms now rooted both within the country at large and the party in particular, social policy and the Social Dimension of the Maastricht Treaty were the obvious targets for Major to attack in the negotiations, thereby pacifying his party at home. The result was the British opt-out from the Social Chapter of the treaty. In fact, even Major's tough stance on the Social Dimension of the Treaty of European Union (TEU) was not enough to satisfy parts of his party and he had to call a confidence motion to get the treaty ratified by the House of Commons (Geddes 1993; Geyer 1997). One can therefore argue that, rather than being ideologically opposed or plain 'awkward', the UK government of the time was not necessarily either, but was simply taking account of the national political situation and pursuing its self-interest, survival in office.

Is Labour's strategy fundamentally different? The level of interaction with the EU and enthusiasm or otherwise for particular policy initiatives is fundamentally dependent on the domestic political situation. There is no doubt that some changes have occurred since 1997, particularly with respect to social policy. Labour did sign up to the Social Chapter, which then became part of the consolidated EU Treaties. With it, Britain is now subject to such legislation as the Works Council Directive and the Working Time Directive. Labour therefore made good on one of its 1997 election promises (Labour Party 1997a). Interestingly, in our interviews with civil servants dealing with EU social policy, a significant number expressed relief at the arrival of the 1997 Labour Government. This was because under the Conservatives they felt that they had no latitude for discussion, bargaining and/or interaction with their EU counterparts over the development of European social policy. With the Conservatives, the central plank of their EU social policy was, 'just say no'.

More fundamentally, within Labour there is no more talk of withdrawal from the EU, as there was in 1983. There are a number of obvious reasons for this. At the EU level, the activities of the Commission President, Jacques Delors (speaking to the Trades Union Congress (TUC) conference in 1988), and the creation of the EU Social Dimension significantly soothed the fears of Labour and the trade unions that the EU was just a capitalist-dominated organisation. Other factors included the role of inter-party tactics. With the Conservatives deeply and publicly split on the issue of Europe, and generally perceived to be 'anti-Europe', it was politically expedient for Labour to present itself as the more pro-EU party. When Labour was elected and immediately ended the social policy opt-out, new directives such as the Working Time Directive demonstrated that Labour was the party that 'brings good things' out of Europe and presented itself as 'being at the heart of Europe' while the Conservatives seek 'isolation'. Also, under Blair, the Labour Party represents itself as both pro-labour and pro-business. Therefore, the EU and its predominately free market ideology are seen as more of an opportunity than a threat. This fits in neatly with the growing recognition that much EU social legislation is based on market-making and enhancing strategies rather than market-regulating ones (Leibfried and Pierson 1996). Lastly, though Labour has become a pro-EU party, there is no evidence to suggest that under the current leadership it is seeking a substantial expansion or alteration of the EU's current social policy development (Broad and Preston 2001).

In fact, even the Liberal Democrats, without doubt the most pro-European of the three major parties, are very sceptical of further integration on social policy. While stating that 'EU legislation in the field of social policy has brought manifest benefits for UK citizens', the party's policy statement goes on to say that:

> The EU should act where required for the smooth functioning of the Internal Market but the main responsibility for social policy should remain with the member states (policy statement on Europe, Liberal Democrat Party website).

So, while the Blair Government has accepted some legislation previously rejected by the Conservatives, mainly done for market-enhancing and internal political reasons (portraying the Conservatives as isolationist), EU–UK social policy interaction must be seen as not just a question of the procedures and institutional arrangements in place, but as dependent on political circumstances at any given time. The evolving and complex interaction between the two levels ebbs and flows over time, altering from extreme intensity to being virtually non-existent.

Do social actors matter?

Up to now all of the actors discussed above are elite central actors, but is there a role for non-elite and regional/local social actors? How do they shape the interaction between the UK and the EU, if indeed they do play a role?

The obvious problem of tracking the impact of the UK social actors in EU–UK social policy interaction is its huge variation and indirect nature (Marks and McAdam 1996; Marks *et al*. 1996). In general, UK social actors, including the trade unions and TUC, play only an indirect role in the creation and implementation of EU social policies in the UK. The larger more internationally oriented trade unions will often have one or possibly two European policy officers. Many smaller unions have none. Most large UK social organisations are aware of European social developments, but do not focus or spend too much time and energy on them. Only the largest employ a European/international officer. The national coordinating organisations, the TUC, National Council for Voluntary Organisations, Women's Commission, Commission for Racial Equality, Local Government International Bureau, etc each employ a small number of European policy staff experts to focus on their particular issues, have links to EU social organisations and put time and effort into pursuing some EU initiatives. However, the costs of influencing the EU level are very high and may have only negligible impacts on the local/regional level. The major exception is in the implementation of the structural funds that will be discussed later.

At the EU level, since the early 1990s there has been an explosive growth of representatives of organised social actors. This was driven by the expansion of the EU and its social agenda and by the desire and support of the European Commission and Parliament to promote a European-wide social dialogue (between capital, labour and the state) and civil dialogue (between the state and various social interests). It reflected the desire to create a political base for Social Europe and a genuine belief that the single market programme should usher in significant developments in social policy to balance the more de-regulatory and market-oriented forces (Martin 1989).

In theory, these European social organisations should be able to organise themselves and become increasingly influential. They have a thriving formal network (the Social Platform which is discussed below) and an extensive informal network, are broadly ideologically similar and pursue similar types of policies. However, these organisational advantages are undermined by a number of problems (Geyer 2000a, 2001). First, the groups are generally (with the exception of the European TUC (ETUC)), relative to most other EU interest groups, young, poor, weak and rely heavily on EU funding. Despite some degree of organisational similarity, there is a clear hierarchy between groups. Groups like the European Women's Lobby or European Youth Forum have budgets over 1 million euros and 10–20 staff members. Meanwhile, other organisations like Eurolink Age (elderly organisation) and Save the Children, for example, have budgets under 100 000 euros and 1–2 staff members. As mentioned above, most groups rely on the EU for funding and are therefore in direct competition with each other over limited resources. Similarly, despite having broad ideological similarities there are a number of political tensions with the EU social actors. For example, a social organisation promoting traditional family life and values might not see eye to eye with a group promoting lesbians' and gays' rights. Thus, while there is broad ideological agreement to champion the cause of the vulnerable, there are disagreements over what constitutes a vulnerable group or which of these should be prioritised.

In response to these weaknesses, the EU and social actors created the Social Platform. Formed in 1996 and largely financed by the Commission, it was intended to act as a central organising forum to enable the social actors to become 'legitimate partners in the public debate on the orientation of European society' (www.socialplatform.org). The Social Platform does organise most (over 30) of the major EU social actors and has run several successful campaigns with the TUC, particularly in relation to the Charter of Fundamental Rights and the EU Constitution. However, despite these successes, the EU social actors remain susceptible to EU disputes (especially with regard to funding), lack a firm base within the EU treaties, exercising 'only a limited degree of influence over the EU policy process and struggling to cooperate with each other on fundamental social issues and political strategies' (Geyer 2001: 478).

Overall, despite sharing general ideological positions and concerns and being well represented within the organisations of EU social actors, relations between UK and EU social actors are not particularly extensive or intensive. On the one hand, the general weakness of EU social actors means that they have little to offer UK national actors and are often hampered by trying to balance a multitude of contradictory member state concerns. On the other hand, UK social actors are often focused on clear local, regional and/or national issues that do not have direct linkages to or implications for EU social actors. Consequently, relations between the two levels are often friendly; most UK social actors were happy to be members of EU social actor networks, but distant. EU policy experts within UK social actors were rarely among the leadership of those organisations. Overall, there is general support for EU–UK social actor interaction, but outside of core policy areas this interaction is very uneven and passive.

There is one notable exception that is worth mentioning, EU regional policy. Here, there are quite distinctive and firm structures in place that, while changeable, are considerably more robust than any other area of social policy. Interestingly, it is also the one area where NGOs, in the form of voluntary organisations, can play quite an important role in the delivery of EU programmes and have significant interaction with both the British Government and political actors at the European level.

The special case of EU regional policy

The European Regional Development Fund (ERDF) and European Social Fund (ESF) form the centrepiece of the EU's regional policy. The value of the funds has grown substantially over its lifetime, so that by the year 2000, the EU spent 32.8 billion euros on regional aid, around a third of its entire budget. After the Common Agricultural Policy, it is the second biggest budget point for the organisation. It is by far the biggest pot of money under what can broadly be defined as 'EU social policy'. However, in national social expenditure this still represents almost small change.

Be that as it may, the amount of money allocated to the UK under structural funds sounds quite impressive; £3.4 billion were earmarked by the EU for the UK between 2000 and 2006. The aim of structural funds is 'to assist areas of the EU that compare unfavourably with the Union average level of prosperity' (Government Office for the North West website). The interesting thing here, and the way the policy differs significantly from most other EU social policies, is that the European Commission has a significant say in where and how that money is spent. For instance, the Commission has the final say on which areas will receive what sort and level of funding, on what type of projects this money can support and the final audit and assessment of the programmes. In many respects it is the lead authority in relation to the structural funds.

Interaction between the European level, the national and the regional and local level of government is extensive. While it is the Commission that runs the Structural Funds Programmes overall, each region designated to receive structural funds has its own programme committee and secretariat to run the programme for its area. The programme committee includes a wide range of representative actors from the central government, local authorities, voluntary sector, private sector, regional development agencies (RDAs), environmental groups and institutions of higher and further education. Each programme area also has a secretariat, which consists of national civil servants based in regional government offices. The secretariat provides administrative support to the programme committee and is often seen as the permanent link between the committee, the Commission and central government. Projects are frequently, but not always, run by local authorities and are often in partnership with the voluntary sector or organisations such as the RDAs. To qualify for support from the ERDF, projects have to promote local/regional economic- and/or infra-structure development.

Clearly, the Structural Funds Programmes involve extensive interaction between the European, national, regional and local levels. The big difference to the interactions in other social policy areas is the structured and institution-alised nature of the arrangements. First and foremost, this is due to the, by EU social policy standards at least, fairly substantial amounts of money involved. With a budget for the UK that runs into several billion pounds it seems inevitable that clearer lines of accountability have developed to ensure that money is spent effectively and accountably. Some commentators argue that the structural funds are really more about the smooth functioning of the single market rather than a 'social' policy (Room 1994). However, if one takes a closer look at the actual working of the funds, one sees a multitude of small, often voluntary organisations involved in the distribution of and work with structural funds to whom this European money makes a real and significant difference. The work they do in the community in terms of training and infrastructure development *is* important and would probably not happen without European money. Structural funds therefore are a significant social policy and are the clearest promoter and indicator of intensive EU–UK social actor interaction (Bachtler and Turock 1997).

Conclusion

While this chapter has been very descriptive in nature, it does demonstrate the difficulty of giving an orderly and clear account of the interaction between the EU and the UK in the sphere of social policy. Clearly, the processes of interaction are extremely complex and constantly changeable. This is the fundamental problem of complexity and can lead one towards a position of relativist uncertainty. If anything can happen, why bother studying it? Nevertheless, there are clear historical legacies and tendencies that make the general outline of EU–UK policy interaction recognisable over longer periods of time. The key problem is finding the balancing point between short-term detailed analyses and long-term historical tendencies. To do this one needs an appropriate theoretical structure that enables one to explore this balance and recognise that this balancing act has similarities throughout the social and even natural worlds. But before this can be done, one needs to explore the general problem of complexity for Europeanisation and UK social policy.

Note

1   Interestingly, an FCO elite claimed that the main advantage of the UK–EU policy relationship relative to other member state–EU policy relationships was that the UK was much more 'joined-up' than the others!

Chapter 2

European integration, UK social policy and the problem of complexity

During one of our many trips to London to interview governmental actors for this book we had an eye-opening experience. It was early in the morning and we were meeting with a high-level civil servant in the Department for Education and Employment. She was very pleasant (as most were) and listened politely as we presented our project and the parameters of the interview. Before we had a chance to ask our first question she blurted out, 'As soon as you understand the larger relationship, you let me know. We have a grip on our particular area, but beyond that we have no idea'. It was a sentiment that was echoed throughout our interviews with governmental and non-governmental actors. It reflected not only the specialisation of one particular departmental actor, but also the much larger problem of interdependence and complexity that confronts public actors.

In this chapter we will argue that this problem of interdependence and complexity runs much deeper than most policy actors and social scientists are willing to admit. As we will demonstrate, early post-World War II (WWII) models and theories of European integration and the welfare state rested on the assumptions of the fundamentally orderly and rational nature of human beings and society. From the 1970s onwards, with the failure of linear social science to capture the fundamental laws of human development, a growing level of inter-national–national human interaction and impact of post-modernist theories and interpretations, social scientists began to look for ways of understanding and dealing with the problem of complexity. Some attempted to reassert different types of orderly frameworks. Others drifted towards the irrationalism of post-modernism and constructivism. Meanwhile, others drifted towards a messy mixture of bounded rationalism and uncertainty. It is this condition of intellectual pluralism that opens the door to something called 'complexity theory' that we will explore in the subsequent chapter.

European integration and the problem of complexity

Complexity has always been a problem for those trying to understand the dynamics of Europeanisation and European integration. From the 1970s when Ernst Haas admitted that one should see the EU as composed 'of infinitely tiered multiple loyalties' (Haas 1970: 635) and Donald Puchala complained that integration researchers were like blind men describing an elephant (Puchala 1972), to the present where Wolfgang Streeck described the European Union (EU) as 'a collection of overlapping functionally specific arrangements for mutual coordination among varying sets of participating countries' (Streeck 1996: 70), and

Philip Schmitter tried to describe it as a 'post-national, unsovereign, polycentric, non-coterminus, neo-medieval arrangement' (Schmitter 1996: 26), complexity has challenged the integration theorist. This recognition of complexity is a core element of the two most influential current approaches to integration: historical institutionalism and multilevel governance. Its influence is so profound that researchers are loath to make larger theoretical propositions and conjectures and continually focus downwards on particular parts of the EU.

Before discussing complexity and Europeanisation directly it is necessary to briefly review the growing theoretical diversification and recognition of complexity in the major theories which surround it: international relations and integration theory and in the concept of globalisation.

International relations: the growth of theoretical diversity and recognition of complexity

As is well known, international relations (IR) theory in the early post-WWII period was dominated by the theory of realism (Morgenthau 1960; Waltz 1979). Realism assumed that nation-states were the primary units at the international level, they were rational utility-maximisers and the international level was an amoral anarchical arena where nation-states competed against one another for economic, political and military advantage. In essence, the system had a clear unchanging order (states in anarchy) that unsurprisingly reflected the experience of the Cold War. Given these assumptions, the international system could be understood from a positivist epistemological and methodological perspective. Nation-states were like balls in motion on a pool table and their behaviour and capabilities were assumed to conform to Newton's laws of motion. They could be rationally calculated and predicted and would tend towards equilibrium (the 'balance of power' concept).

By the 1970s with the collapse of the Bretton Woods economic system, growth of transnational corporations and cooling of the Cold War, interdependence or regime theorists began to emerge (Keohane and Nye 1977; Krasner 1983). They stressed that the international system was not wholly anarchical, international actors had emerged and were increasingly important and the actions and interests of national actors could be reshaped by the 'web of interdependence' or 'regimes'. These theorists often tried to adhere to the positivist tradition. However, the 'bounded rationality' of the main actors, the growing number and complexity of the key actors and the uncertain developments made a strict adherence to this tradition increasingly difficult. The international arena could no longer be understood as uniformly orderly and therefore analysed through purely reductionist and parsimonious strategies.

In the 1980s and 1990s, both realists and interdependence/regime theorists were criticised by reflectivist theories. These theories incorporate a broad range of perpectives from critical theory and feminism, to post-modernism and post-structuralism (Ashley 1986; Walker 1993; Checkel 1998). Reflectivists emphasised that much of international relations (and realism in particular) were ideological constructs created by the dominant powers in the international system. Neither the actors nor the system were inherently rational, and what was deemed to be rational in one time or context may vary in another time or context. Many reflectivists adopted anti-naturalist and anti-foundationalist positions, arguing that human experience was inherently distinctive from natural phenomena and that there could be no certain epistemological foundations for claims to fundamental human truths. Reality was what one made of it.

From the early 1990s, constructivists (Onuf 1989; Adler 1997; Wendt 1999) attempted to 'build a bridge between these two traditions' (Wendt 1992: 394) by emphasising ontological and epistemological openness. Not surprisingly, despite these bridge-building efforts, both rationalists and reflectivists have continued to exclude and ignore each other while clinging to the certainty of their orderly or disorderly ontological/epistemological claims. For example, rationalists attempted to co-opt constructivism by arguing that, 'rationalism ... and constructivism now provide the major points of contestation for international relations scholarship' (Katzenstein *et al.* 1998: 646) and exclude reflectivism by stressing that:

> [it] *denies ... the use of evidence to adjudicate between truth claims ...* [it] *falls clearly outside of the social science enterprise, and in IR research it risks becoming self-referential and disengaged from the world, protests to the contrary notwithstanding* (Katzenstein *et al.* 1998: 678).

On the other side, reflectivists have complained that social constructivism goes too far in a rationalist direction, accepting many of the major constructs such as the primacy of nation-states and drifting towards a positivist methodology (Smith 2001a). Thus, despite good intentions, the bridge-building strategy of constructivism appears to have stalled.

The short rise and fall of 'hard' globalisation

Out of this complex theoretical debate emerged the real and perceived impact of globalisation. Emerging out of the rapid development of international capital markets in the 1970s, 1980s and 1990s, the revival of neo-liberal economic policy in the USA and UK (Reagan and Thatcher 'revolutions'), and the economic difficulties following the collapse of the Bretton Woods system, globalisation was seen as a new hegemonic economic force which would empower capital, undermine state powers, and force all advanced industrial countries (let alone Third World countries) to pursue neo-liberal economic policies, abandon welfare states and create a destructive competition between national social and environmental systems of regulation (Ohmae 1990, 1995). However, as political and academic debates raged in the 1990s, it became increasingly obvious that the impact and development of globalisation was more complex than the early thinkers/ideologues had assumed. Summarised nicely in the work of Paul Hirst and Grahame Thompson (Hirst and Thompson 1996), observers began to note that despite growing economic regionalisation within the First World, the Third World was being left out of the process. Despite greater capital mobility and the internationalisation of production, general trade flows and patterns remained remarkably stable. Despite the collapse of traditional Keynesian fiscal policy, active monetary, regional and labour market policies remained viable. Finally, despite significant pressures on taxation levels and welfare regimes in advanced industrial states, taxation levels had remained remarkably stable (Swank 1998) and welfare state expenditure had actually grown slightly during the period (Hay 2001). Not surprisingly, given this growing body of 'limited globalisation', the focus began to shift from seeing globalisation as a hard 'hegemonic force' to a softer 'interactive influence' on national systems (Axtmann 1998; Geyer 1996; Prakash and Hart 1999; Sykes *et al*. 2001). By the end of the 1990s, globalisation became much more uncertain, variable, complex and interdependent.

European integration theory: from simple to complex interaction

European integration (EI) theory mirrored much of the post-WWII development of IR theory (Rosamond 2000; Chryssochoou 2001). In the 1950s and 1960s, the core European integration debate involved intergovernmentalists, who saw the EU as an intergovernmental extension of a fundamentally realist international order, and functionalists/neo-functionalists, who saw the early EU as possessing the ability to functionally reshape the realist international order (at least within Western Europe). During these years, debates raged over the degree to which early EU policy developments were determined by intergovernmental bargains or functional spillover. The fates of the theories were tied to the success or failure of the integration process. When it succeeded, neo-functionalists boasted. When it faltered, intergovernmentalists exulted.

Following a period of stagnation in the 1970s, when many integration theorists drifted to other areas of research, integration theory revived in the 1980s and 1990s with the revival of integration through the Single European Market project. New theories, linked to the earlier ones, began to recognise the more complex and uncertain nature of European integration (Taylor 1983). Andrew Moravcsik carried the torch for intergovermentalists. However, even his concept of liberal intergovernmentalism recognised the importance of complex institutional dynamics (Moravcsik 1993). Others (Tranholm-Mikkelsen 1991) held on to a modified neo-functionalism. Both theories were brought together by multilevel governance theorists (Hooghe and Marks 2001) who argued that the EU was composed of 'overlapping competencies of among multiple levels of governments and the interaction of political actors across those levels' (Marks *et al*. 1996: 41).

Despite this increasing recognition of complexity, or because of it, reflectivist and constructivist works came late to EI theory, only beginning to emerge in the late 1990s (Jørgensen 1997; Checkel 1998, 1999; Diez 1999; Christiansen *et al*. 2001). Again, similar to the experience in IR theory, constructivists saw themselves as 'establishing a middle ground' (Christiansen *et al*. 2001: 8) between rationalist and reflectivist paradigms. Unsurprisingly, they came under fire from both sides of the debate. On the one hand, reflectivists complained that it was:

> *Far more 'rationalist' in character than 'reflectivist'; indeed I would go so far as to say that social constructivism in its dominant* [mainly North American] *form is very close to the neoliberalist wing of the rationalist paradigm* (Smith 2001b: 191).

On the other hand, rationalists argued that:

All this [philosophical speculation] *distracts constructivists from the only element truly essential to social science: the vulnerability of conjectures to some sort of empirical disconfirmation* (Moravcsik 2001: 186).

Moreover, Mark Pollack, echoing the conclusions of Katzenstein *et al.* (1998) in IR theory, argued that EI theory must accept 'broader ontologies', but:

we must necessarily fall back on careful empirical testing ... as the ultimate, and indeed the only, standard of what constitutes 'good work' and what constitutes support for one approach or another (Pollack 2001: 236).

Just like IR, EI theory was divided into two opposing poles and a struggling bridging strategy.

Europeanisation: the baby brother of globalisation

Europeanisation as a marketable academic concept emerged on the back of the aforementioned success of European integration and impact of globalisation in the 1990s. For many, particularly in the early 1990s, it became the regional extension of the globalisation debate. As Gamble notes, 'it is most widely understood as the penetration of the European dimension into the national arena', but after this rather straightforward assertion, 'the agreement tends to stop' (Gamble 2001). In the context of welfare issues, since the international economy was globalising and putting pressure on national welfare states, the EU had to either embrace and enhance this development or build walls to protect the distinctive importance of 'Social Europe'. These debates were particularly visible in the areas of EU social policy and European welfare state research (Leibfried and Pierson 1995; Rhodes 1996; Geyer 2000b).

However, again similar to the fate of globalisation, Europeanisation became a much more subtle, complex and interactive concept as the 1990s progressed. Despite the growing influence of the EU in a multitude of policy areas, national policy regimes remained remarkably distinctive. The research focus began to shift from how Europe was shaping national policy regimes to how national regimes were interacting with and adjusting to EU developments. Numerous nationally and comparatively oriented works began to emerge to explore this detailed interaction (Esping-Andersen 1996; Bonoli *et al.* 2000; Ferrera and Rhodes 2000; Leibfried and Obinger 2000; Cowles *et al.* 2001; Knill 2001; Sykes *et al.* 2001).

One of the most comprehensive and systematic of these works was developed by Claudio Radaelli (2001). He argued that there were at least four possible national outcomes to the processes of Europeanisation:

- **inertia:** where no change occurs at the national level
- **adaptation/absorption:** where EU policy is absorbed by the national level, thus implying some degree of domestic policy change as a result of European level impulses
- **transformation:** where EU developments induce a fundamental shift in the existing national policy framework
- **retrenchment:** where national policy approaches are augmented by European dynamics.

Moreover, these outcomes were caused by a variable combination of 'vertical' and 'horizontal' Europeanisation. Vertical forces include 'hard' laws and regulations, such as market-regulating measures, where there is a direct requirement for member states to adapt to EU level requirements. Horizontal forces are 'soft' laws and indirect processes of change, such as the open method of coordination or the growth of EU norms, where there is no direct pressure to conform to EU policy.

However, like most of the other authors working on Europeanisation, Radaelli could identify some of the general aspects of Europeanisation but freely admitted that there was no general pattern or direction to the process. Europeanisation was a multilevel process where historical pathways, institutions, member states and economic and social actors all played variable roles over time. These conclusions were mirrored by two other major works on Europeanisation. In his impressive book on the Europeanisation of national administrations, Christoph Knill concluded that:

> *the form, logic and scope of everything that happens within this macro-institutional range* [of national administrative traditions] *varies with European policies, domestic interest constellations, beliefs and expectations as well as institutional opportunity structures* (Knill 2001: 227).

Meanwhile, in the conclusion to their path breaking edited volume, Maria Green Cowles and Thomas Risse argued that:

> *Europeanization does not result in the homogenization of domestic structures. Member states face varying degrees of adaptational pressures to the 'regulatory patchwork' of EU rules and regulations. Different factors restrain or facilitate their adaptation to these Europeanization pressures. Yet, the transformation of domestic strctures takes place all the same, oftentimes in rather fundamental ways* (Cowles *et al.* 2001: 236).

In essence, in the new millennium, simple positions regarding the costs and benefits of the EU and Europeanisation were being buried under a mountain of more subtle and interactive analyses. European integration and Europeanisation had become ripe for some form of complexity theory.

The British welfare state and the problem of complexity

Similar to international relations and European integration, the study of the British political system and welfare state have also gone through a complexity shift in the latter half of the 20th century. In the 1950s and 1960s, theories of British politics and the state revolved around the ideal of the 'Westminster model' which emphasised centralised power in the hands of the core executive and Parliament with a supposedly apolitical civil service carrying out the democratic will of the people. Lines of authority, power and legitimacy were clear and rational. Likewise, the Beveridge welfare state was seen as the progressive culmination of the development of Marshallian civil, political and social rights. Rationally correcting the limitations of the market, the welfare state would continuously improve fundamental living standards (Marshall 1964; Fraser 1973).

However, linked to the poor economic performance of the British economy and the perception of an increasingly burdensome welfare state, during the 1970s a variety of potent critics began to question the usefulness and coherence of the Westminster model and traditional welfare state. From the left, some argued that the expansion of the welfare state was incompatible with the continued functioning of capitalism (Miliband 1973; Gough 1979). The right countered with the 'overload thesis' (King 1976; Brittan 1977) that stressed that the welfare state was part of a larger problem of state expansion in the post-WWII period. As the state became increasingly responsible for social outcomes, demands expanded exponentially and overloaded the political system, increased 'ungovernability', fomented a fiscal crisis of the state and created a dependency culture among the population. With the rise of Margaret Thatcher and success of the Conservative Party, the overload thesis appeared to have won the day.

This perception of overload and inefficiency coalesced easily with the growing debate over the impact of globalisation and Europeanisation. Particularly for the right, global economic development and pressure required states to abandon traditional forms of welfare and adopt more market-oriented approaches. Economic success and survival depended on it. Likewise, the emerging European single market had to concentrate on enhancing these competitive pressures and market forces if Europe was to survive in the increasingly competitive global system. As Margaret Thatcher famously warned in her attack on European social policy in 1988, 'we have not rolled back the frontiers of the state to see them re-imposed from Brussels'.

Nevertheless, despite the polemical success of the overload thesis and the growth of globalisation and Europeanisation, welfare states refused to collapse or converge. In Britain, as many commentators noted (Krieger 1986), the radical anti-statist polemics of the Thatcher Governments were not matched by similar policies. The British welfare state was restructured, but not radically reduced. Modes of welfare delivery have been altered (particularly with the rise of 'new public management': *see* Newman 2000), but 'there has been no wholesale transfer of state welfare provision into the private sector (with the partial exception of housing)' (Pierson 1999: 157). More broadly, within the advanced industrial countries there has been no significant decline in welfare state expenditure or significant convergence of welfare state structures (Goodin *et al.* 1999; Cochrane *et al.* 2001). Moreover, as discussed earlier, the EU has not radically undermined existing national welfare states, forced them to significantly converge or created a new European-level welfare state. Out of these debates and the rise of post-modernist social theory emerged more subtle and broadranging interpretations of British politics and, the welfare state that tried to go beyond the traditional left–right debates. These included the development of the governance approach in British politics and, most influentially, the concept of the 'third way' by Anthony Giddens. Due to its political impact on the welfare state and left more generally, we must take some time to more thoroughly discuss the third way.

The 'third way'

Defining the 'third way' is a notoriously slippery problem. The current use of the term 'third way' is often poorly defined, obfuscated by political opportunism and complicated by distinctive national interpretations.[1] Politically, the concept clearly fulfilled the needs of 'modernisers' in leftist parties looking for an intellectual and theoretical justification for shifting their parties towards the political centre. With the success of the Clinton administration in 1992 and 1996, the Blair victory in 1997 and the Schroeder victory in Germany, the 'third way' became an influential and widely discussed political strategy and theory. Intellectually, the modern concept of the 'third way' has generated a significant discussion (Powell 1999; Giddens 2000) and is based strongly on two key books by Giddens, *Beyond Left and Right: the future of radical politics* (1994) and *The Third Way: the renewal of social democracy* (1998).

Beyond Left and Right was Giddens' most thorough attempt to create a wide-ranging modern philosophy and strategy for the left. Its strength lay in the concept of 'manufactured risk/uncertainty'. Following in the footsteps of a number of post-modern authors and sociological intellectual traditions, Giddens argued that, 'the world we live in today is not one subject to tight human mastery' (Giddens 1994: 4). This is not due to the complexity of nature or the failure of humankind to master it, but due to 'our conscious intrusion into our own history and our interventions into nature' (Giddens 1994: 78). For Giddens, due to the development of industrialisation, globalisation, a post-traditional social order and the rise of 'social reflexivity' (Beck 1992), uncertainty and risk can no longer be externalised to natural occurrences, but are more and more a product of human action and awareness. In other words, despite the hopes of the 'enlightenment', where humanity would increasingly entrench its dominance over natural and social conditions, the very pursuit of this dominance had led to the creation of human-manufactured uncertainty and risk that altered the fundamental framework of our relationship to the natural world and human social development.

Much of the remainder of the book focuses on the implications of manufactured uncertainty/risk. For example, given no 'tight human mastery' over the world and a reflexive society, then the authority and certainty of tradition, science, experts and bureaucratic organisations must be questioned and re-interpreted. For Giddens, one had to be careful not to allow this re-interpretation to lead to a 'new medievalism' of back-to-nature green movements (Giddens 1994: 79), a post-modernist attraction to Nietzschian nihilism (Giddens 1994: 252) or a reassertion of 'fundamentalism' (Giddens 1994: 6). Nevertheless, recognising the inherently uncertain nature of human existence and the manufactured nature of those uncertainties and risks was essential to establishing a viable and radical new theory and strategy for the left.

The need to recognise and respond to manufactured risk/uncertainty lies at the heart of Giddens' explanation for and solution to the current crisis of social democracy. For Giddens, the early appeal and fundamental weakness of Marxism was that it rested on the belief that humanly created problems must be humanly resolvable and, consequently, that it had found the fundamental direction of human evolution. This basic belief in the ability of revolutionary (later, technocratic) elites to direct and understand human economic and social interaction manifested itself in the planned economies under communism and the belief in planning in the advanced industrial economies in the early post-WWII period. For Giddens, this 'cybernetic model' was 'reasonably effective as a means of generating economic development in conditions of simple modernization' (Giddens 1994: 66). However, as societies and economies become more complicated and reflexive, the cybernetic model became increasingly dysfunctional. As Giddens wrote:

> *A modern economy can tolerate, and prosper under, a good deal of central planning only so long as certain conditions hold – so long as it is primarily a national economy; social life is segmentalized rather than penetrated extensively by globalizing influences; and the degree of institutional reflexivity is not high. As these circumstances alter, Keynesianism falters and Soviet-type economies stagnate* (Giddens 1994: 67).

Consequently, with the collapse of the Soviet Union in 1989 and the difficulties of social democracy in Sweden in the late 1980s, often seen as the most developed social democratic society, socialism lost its radical edge and fell back on a static defence of the welfare state. Meanwhile, neo-liberals, espousing the ability of the unfettered market to solve both economic and social ills, 'appropriated the future-oriented radicalism which was once the hallmark of the bolder forms of socialist thinking' (Giddens 1994: 73).

In order to bring radicalism back to the left Giddens explored the implications of manufactured risk/uncertainty on a variety of policy arenas, particularly the welfare state. He argued that the left had to abandon its traditional defence of the welfare state and replace them with ideas of 'positive welfare'. For Giddens, 'the welfare state cannot survive in its existing form' (Giddens 1994: 174). Like Keynesian economic ideas, the welfare state performed well under conditions of simple modernisation:

> *in which 'industriousness' and paid work remained central to the social system; where class relations were closely linked to communal forms; where the nation-state was strong and even in some respects further developing its sovereign powers; and where risk could still be treated largely as external and to be coped with by quite orthodox programmes of social insurance. None of these conditions holds in the same way in conditions of intensifying globalization and social reflexivity* (Giddens 1994: 149).

Consequently, the attempt by the welfare state to combat stable external risks, for example unemployment insurance, may lead to contradictory outcomes such as welfare dependency rather than encouraging a return to work. Thus, the left defence of the welfare state is ultimately doomed to failure. Without abandoning the 'providentialism', that history has a particular direction, of the leftist programme, accepting the new conditions of manufactured risk/uncertainty and reforming its thinking, particularly in regard to its last defensive stronghold (the welfare state), the left will never regain its historical radicalism.

The Third Way, a remarkably wide-selling book that summarised and popularised his thinking in *Beyond Left and Right*, extended the third way to a wide variety of policy implications. Regarding the welfare state, Giddens again argued that the third way charted a middle path between the antagonism towards state activities by liberals, and an uncritical faith in it by socialists. The current welfare state 'isn't geared up to cover new-style risks such as those concerning technological change, social exclusion or the accelerating proportion of one-parent households' (Giddens 1998: 116). It needs to adopt a 'positive welfare' approach and transform itself into a 'social investment state'. A positive welfare approach implies that the welfare state needs to help combat the classical external risks and promote society's ability to adapt to manufactured risks. In order to do this it needs to become 'dynamic and responsive to wider social trends', 'promote risk-taking by individuals' and 'invest in human capital wherever possible' (Giddens 1998: 117). Consequently, according to Giddens:

> positive welfare would replace each of Beveridge's negatives with a positive:
> in place of Want, autonomy; not Disease but active health; instead of
> Ignorance, education, as a continuing part of life; rather than Squalor, well-
> being; and in place of Idleness, initiative (Giddens 1998: 128).

As is well known, the third way generated an enormous amount of comment and criticism. Some argued that it was 'an amorphous political project, difficult to pin down and lacking direction' (Giddens 2000: 22), others (Ryan 1999; Driver and Martell 2000) that it was merely the reassertion of an earlier British tradition of New Liberalism. The traditional left (Hall 1998; Lafointaine 1998) argued that it was a rationalisation for a shift to the right while academics and politicians in Continental Europe (Levy 1999; Lightfoot 1999) argued that it was fundamentally an Anglo-Saxon project that 'was of little use to societies that are further along the road to social justice and more comprehensive welfare provision' (Giddens 2000: 24).

   Basically, all of these critics wanted the third way to be more specific, linear and predictive. Whether arguing that the third way was not distinctive enough from historical precedents, was too vague, was a rationalisation and/or did not fit their particular models, all of these critics were trying to force Giddens to justify his more post-modern, contingent and reflexive framework. Giddens responded to these criticisms from a predominantly linear position, i.e. that the third way was a new type of order that could be opposed to earlier forms of order.

   For example, in responding to his continental critics he argued that in spite of the distinctiveness of most European socialist parties and welfare state regimes there is 'a single broad stream of third way thinking, to which the various parties and governments are contributing' (Giddens 2000: 31). Hence, despite their differences they are all part of a similar linear trend or process. The third way developed so early and clearly in the US and UK because both 'experienced neoliberal government in "full-blooded form"' (Giddens 2000: 32). This made the left in the US and UK more willing to question traditional orthodoxies and shift towards the third way. Moreover, argued Giddens, those social democratic countries that appear to be the most traditional, particularly Scandinavia, 'are likely to be more vulnerable to the changes now happening than countries "further back" on the welfare scale' (Giddens 2000: 34).

   On the other hand, a number of critics from different perspectives argued that, fundamentally, the third way was primarily an attempt to reassert a new linear order. As Nikolas Rose pointed out, the third way 'describes the present in epochal terms, implying that there is only one right way to understand and respond to the real changes occurring in our world' (Rose 1999: 490). Consequently, they (referring to Giddens and Will Hutton):

> *draw a diagram of history in which a single axis of time catches up all corners of the globe into its current and drags all along its wake* ... [all must] *become modern or face the destiny of the obsolete – the scrap heap of history* (Rose 1999: 471).

Ted Benton further clarifies this point by stressing that, 'despite his disclaimers, Giddens himself remains committed to key elements of a linear, developmental view of history' (Benton 1999: 44). Most influentially, Ralf Dahrendorf attacked the 'authoritarian streak' in the third way:

> *The great liberation of the revolution of 1989 was that it ended the dominance of ideological thought systems. There are no longer even first, second and third worlds, only varieties of attempts to cope with economic, social and political needs. The Third Way presupposes a more Hegelian view of the world. It forces its adherents to define themselves in relation to others, rather than by their own peculiar combination of ideas; and the others have to be invented, even caricatured for the purpose. The point about an open world is that there are not just two or three ways. There are ... 101 ways, which is to say, an indefinite number* (Dahrendorf 1999).

Interestingly, despite mentioning Dahrendorf's intimations of an 'authoritarian streak' in the third way, Giddens did not reply to the criticism in Giddens (2000). This is very telling because it is the most fundamental criticism from a complexity perspective. Giddens' entire theory rests on an understanding of manufactured uncertainty/risk. This implies that no individual or elite actor is capable of understanding the path of history in a linear sense. However, despite his protestations, the third way implies that it understands the next phase of human development and thus can and should control that development. Thus, if the world has changed (due to globalisation, reflexivity, etc) and the third way is capable of understanding that shift, then the third way can become the new 'radical' historical order which saves the left and restores it to its position at the forefront of history.

Given this combination of policy openness and underlying order and control, one can easily see why the third way would be so appealing to New Labour. In political terms it allowed the party to justify its abandoning of unpopular traditional strategies under the veneer of a new vaguely defined order. In policy areas, it legitimated the ability of the Blair Government to pursue seemingly decentralising policies in a context of centralised audit and control. The most blaring examples occur with the welfare state, particularly in the education and health sectors, where the calls for local control and autonomy have been strangled by the centralising flurry of continued 'new managerialism' (Walsh 1995) and an intensified audit culture (Rouse and Smith 1999).

The possibilities of policy transfer theory

Clearly, the implications of the above discussion are that the Europeanisation–British welfare state relationship is a prime site for complex and contingent processes and outcomes. Both Europeanisation and the British welfare state are composed of evolving complex institutions adapting, learning and adjusting to a contingent multitiered political–economic arena: multilevel governance meets the third way.

Academic works that attempt to explore this relationship, or other EU–member state policy relationships, often fall back on a very thick descriptive type of analysis. It isn't that this type of methodological approach is wrong given the problems of complexity and interdependent contingency. However, one is always left with a sense of incompleteness or even failure, seen from the perspective of a linear framework. Detailed studies are created, great effort is made, but the results are only partially relevant to other areas/cases and will certainly change over time. Rather than creating general rules with predictive capabilities, the researcher gains only a sense of the continually evolving process and recognises that this is only partially relevant to other areas and the future direction of the policy. From an orderly linear perspective, the researcher is stuck like Sisyphus, doomed to endlessly describe a process that never reaches its goal.

Not surprisingly, few theoreticians are willing to delve into this mire of contingency and uncertainty. One notable exception is the work of policy transfer theorists. Policy transfer theory emerged in the mid-1990s particularly in relation to the study of policy transfer between the USA and UK (Rose 1993; Dolowitz and Marsh 1996; Stone 1999). Policy transfer (PT) theorists concentrated on examining the processes through which policies were transferred and/or learned from one policy, institutional or political arena to another. In general, these works concentrated on policy transfer as a voluntary 'learning' process between independent states. However, PT theory could be applied to learning between different levels of government and in coercive situations as well. PT theorists argued that policy transfer could lead to policy convergence, but that the transfer of policies was not a simple linear process and that it often led to unintended results and consequences due to the different nature of the national policy arenas.

Interestingly, despite its obvious implications, PT theorists only recently (with the early exception of Rose (1993)) began using their concepts to describe EU policy dynamics (Bomberg and Peterson 2000; Radaelli 2001). For these theorists, recent development of EU policy transfers have been driven by:

> *exchanges between national authorities who share a common concern to solve policy problems, as well as causal understandings and technical expertise. In essence EU policy transfer is a pro-active – and only rarely coercive – approach to the Europeanization of public policy* (Bomberg and Peterson 2000: 7).

From this perspective, policy transfer strategies have evolved because member states have become increasingly dissatisfied with traditional EU policy methods. The growth of open methods of coordination, mainstreaming, etc are clear indicators of the success of this new approach which provides a range of substantial political and policy benefits, such elite learning and depoliticised policy interaction. It may also promote convergence. However, PT theorists are quick to emphasise, the growth of EU policy transfer does not imply convergence. As mentioned above, learning can have both convergent and divergent outcomes. Moreover, policy transfer does not replace all policy dynamics. It is a growing area, but one which interacts with, rather than dominates traditional policy methods.

In general, policy transfer theory is not dissimilar from multilevel governance (MLG) theory or the general theoretical concepts of Anthony Giddens' 'third way', particularly in terms of their emphasis on the complexity and openness of the evolution of policies. Moreover, I would argue very strongly that MLG- and PT-based researchers have produced very good descriptions of the EU policy process. However, are they really scientific theories in the traditional sense? They are not very parsimonious, admitting as they do that many other factors are at play in EU policy development. They do not explain causality very well, seeing multiple influences on particular outcomes. They are not predictive, emphasising historical openness. Moreover, they do not lead to universal rules; each case has its own dynamics. Fundamentally, it looks as if they will never fulfil traditional scientific criteria. But, should they?

Conclusion

If one steps back and looks at the larger process of theorising about international relations, European integration, the welfare state and policy interaction, one finds a remarkable similarity in theoretical developments. At the same time as social life in advanced industrial countries has become more complex, theoretical positions have increasingly represented these new experiences. Moreover, with the growing ease of communication between societies and academic communities, ideas from one field have rapidly influenced those in other fields. In essence, all of these areas are in the process of confronting the problem of complexity. The core weakness for these theories in addressing the complexity problem is that due to the problem's fundamental nature, the theories tend to revert back to a traditional linear scientific framework to try and solve the problem. The difficulty is that from a traditional scientific framework, complexity can never resolved. It is always a problem. However, since the early 20th century a new scientific framework or paradigm, complexity theory, has been emerging out of the physical and natural sciences. This new framework does not solve the problem of complexity, but allows us to understand it in new and exciting ways. Introducing and exploring this new theory will be the object of Chapter 3.

Note

[1] Recognising the confusion which surrounded the term, Giddens stated that, 'the term third way is of no particular significance ... I make use of it here to refer to social democratic renewal' (Giddens 1998: VII).

What is complexity theory?

What is complexity theory? How and when did it emerge? Is it a hot new academic fad like globalisation or the end of history, or is it something more profound? To begin to answer these questions we need to jump back a few centuries and briefly discuss the emergence of what is variously labelled as the Newtonian or linear paradigm. For reasons that will become clear, we have called it the paradigm of order.

The paradigm of order

Although it has been said thousands of times before, it bears repeating, the Enlightenment was an astounding time for Europe. Relatively stagnant and weak and intellectually repressed by the Church during the so-called Dark Ages, intellectual energies released by the Renaissance came to fruition in the Enlightenment. During this time, Europe was reborn and became the centre of an intellectual, technical and economic transformation. It had an enormous impact on the way life is viewed at all levels from the mundane to the profound. Science was liberated from centuries of control by religious stipulations and blind trust in ancient philosophies. René Descartes (1596–1650) and, slightly later, Sir Isaac Newton (1642–1727) set the scene. The former advocated rationalism while the latter unearthed a wondrous collection of fundamental laws. A flood of other discoveries in diverse fields such as magnetism, electricity, astronomy and chemistry soon followed, injecting a heightened sense of confidence in the power of reason to tackle any situation. The growing sense of human achievement led the famous author and scientist Alexander Pope to poeticise, 'Nature, and Nature's laws lay hid in night. God said "Let Newton be!" And all was light'. Later, the 18th century French scientist and author of *Celestial Mechanics* Pierre Simon de Laplace (1749–1827) carried the underlying determinism of the Newtonian framework to its logical conclusion by arguing that, 'if at one time, we knew the positions and motion of all the particles in the universe, then we could calculate their behaviour at any other time, in the past or future'.

The subsequent phenomenal success of the industrial revolution in the 18th and 19th centuries, which was based on this new scientific approach, created a high degree of confidence in the power of human reason to tackle any physical situation. By the late 19th and early 20th century many scientists believed that few surprises remained to be discovered. For the American Nobel Laureate, Albert Michelson (1852–1931), 'the future truths of physical science are to be looked for in the sixth place of decimals' (Horgan 1996: 19). From that time onwards, physicists would merely be filling in the cracks in human knowledge. More fundamentally, the assumption and expectation was that over time the orderly nature of all phenomena would eventually be revealed to the human mind. Science became the search for hidden order.

By and large, that vision of the universe survived well into the 20th century. In 1996 John Horgan, a senior writer at *Scientific American*, published a best-selling book entitled *The End of Science* which argued that since science was linear and all the major discoveries had been made, then real science had come to an end. All that was left was 'ironic science' which:

> *does not make any significant contributions to knowledge itself. Ironic science is thus less akin to science in the traditional sense than to literary criticism – or to philosophy* (Horgan 1996: 31).

Similarly, the eminent biologist and Pulitzer prize winner, Edward O Wilson argued in his bestselling book *Consilience* (1999) that all science should be unified in a fundamentally linear framework based on physics:

> *The central idea of the consilience world view is that all tangible phenomena, from the birth of stars to the workings of social institutions, are based on material processes that are ultimately reducible, however long and tortuous the sequences, to the laws of physics* (Wilson 1999: 291).

The linear view of the world prospered not only in the sciences, but in the fundamental nature of Western social and political life.

To simplify drastically, the paradigm of order was founded on four golden rules:

- **order:** given causes lead to known effects at all times and places
- **reductionism:** the behaviour of a system could be understood, clockwork fashion, by observing the behaviour of its parts. There are no hidden surprises; the whole is the sum of the parts, no more and no less
- **predictability:** once global behaviour is defined, the future course of events could be predicted by application of the appropriate inputs to the model
- **determinism:** processes flow along orderly and predictable paths that have clear beginnings and rational ends.

From these golden rules a simple picture of reality emerged as shown in Figure 3.1.

Given the golden rules and picture of reality, several expectations emerged:

- over time as human knowledge increases, phenomena will shift from the disorderly to the orderly side
- knowledge equals order. Hence, greater knowledge equals greater order
- with greater knowledge/order humans can increasingly predict and control more and more phenomena
- there is an endpoint to phenomena and hence knowledge.

The orderly paradigm worked remarkably well and was conspicuous by incredible leaps in technological, scientific and industrial achievements. Science became orderly and hierarchical with clear divisions that manifested themselves

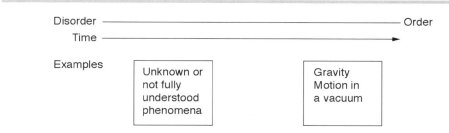

Figure 3.1 Phenomena in the paradigm of order.

in the departmentalised evolution of modern universities and in a hierarchy of sciences. As the Nobel prize-winning physicist (though he won the award for chemistry) Ernest Rutherford famously said, 'All science is either physics or stamp collecting'. Not surprisingly, success in these areas had a profound effect on attitudes in all sectors of human activity, spreading well beyond the disciplines covered by the original discoveries.

Ripples of doubt

Certainty and predictability for all, the hallmarks of an orderly frame of mind, were too good to last. Fissures had existed for some time; even Isaac Newton and Christiaan Huygens in the 17th century couldn't agree on something as fundamental as the nature of light (is it a particle or a wave?). These difficulties bubbled under the surface of acceptable scientific discourse and the expanding university arenas. They were often seen as unimportant phenomena that would be resolved by the next wave of emerging fundamental laws. However, by the early 20th century they could no longer be ignored. Henri Poincaré (1854–1912), the supreme physicist of his age, was one of the first to voice disquiet about some contemporary scientific beliefs. He advanced ideas that pre-dated chaos theory by some 70 years (Coveney and Highfield 1995: 169). Later, Einstein's (1879–1955) theory of relativity, Neils Bohr's (1885–1962) contribution to quantum mechanics, Erwin Schrödinger's (1887–1961) quantum measurement problem, Werner Heisenberg's (1901–1976) uncertainty principle and Paul AM Dirac's (1902–1984) work on quantum field theory all played a decisive role in pushing conventional wisdom beyond the Newtonian limits that enclosed it centuries before. These scientists, all Nobel laureates, set in motion a process that eventually transformed attitudes in many other disciplines.[1]

The new discoveries did not disprove Newton. Essentially, they revealed that not all phenomena were orderly, reducible, predictable and/or determined. For example, no matter how hard classical physicists tried they could not fit the dualistic nature of light as both a wave and a particle into the orderly classical system. Heisenberg's uncertainty principle, which shows that one can either know the momentum or position of a subatomic particle, but not both at the same time, presents an obvious problem for the orderly paradigm. Or, the paradox of Schrodinger's Cat experiment, which demonstrated the distinctive nature of quantum probability, again broke the fundamental boundaries of the former order. What this meant was that even at the most fundamental level some phenomena do conform to the classical framework, others do not. With this, the boundaries of the classical paradigm were cast asunder. Gravity continued to function and linear mechanics continued to work, but it could no longer claim to be universally applicable to all physical phenomena. It had to live alongside phenomena and theories that were essentially *probabilistic*. They do not conform to the four golden rules associated with linearity: order, reductionism, predictability and determinism. Causes and effects are not linked, the whole is not simply the sum of the parts; *emergent properties* often appear seemingly out of the blue, taking the system apart does not reveal much about its global behaviour, and the related processes do not steer the systems to inevitable and distinct ends (*see* Figure 3.2).

Given these non-linear phenomena and non-adherence to the golden rules of order, new expectations were necessary for this expanding paradigm:

* over time human knowledge may increase, but phenomena will not necessarily shift from the disorderly to the orderly
* knowledge does not always equal order. Greater knowledge may mean the increasing recognition of the limits of order/knowledge
* greater knowledge does not necessarily impart greater prediction and control. Greater knowledge may indicate increasing limitations to prediction and control
* there is no universal structure/endpoint to phenomena/knowledge.

It is important to note that the shift in scientific analysis from utter certainty to considerations of probability was not accepted lightly. Schrodinger had originally designed his cat experiment as a way of eliminating the duality problem! The sea change radiated slowly outwards from quantum mechanics' domain of subatomic particles. Naturally, there was a wide schism between the exclusive niches occupied by leading particle physicists and mathematicians, on the one hand, and the rest of the scientific community, on the other. High specialisation meant that even scholars involved in the same discipline were not immediately aware of discoveries being made by their colleagues. Moreover, the language of science itself became almost unintelligible beyond a select circle of specialists. In any case, their intriguing speculations were not thought at first to be of everyday concern. Nevertheless, uncertainty was eventually recognised as an inevitable feature of some situations. In effect, the envelope of orderly science was expanded to add complex phenomena, also know as *complex systems*, to those already in place.

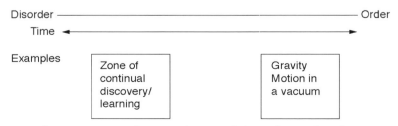

Figure 3.2 **Phenomena in the paradigms of disorder and order.**

Complex systems in an abiotic world

Once the door was open to probability and uncertainty, a new wave of scientists began studying phenomena that had previously been ignored or considered secondary or uninteresting, Rutherford's 'stamp-collecting' activities.[2] Weather patterns, fluid dynamics and Boolean networks were just three of the areas that saw the growing acceptance of non-linear complex phenomena and systems. For example, one of the earliest people to conceptualise and model a non-linear complex system was an American meteorologist, Edward Lorenz (Gleick 1988). Lorenz developed a computer program for modelling weather systems in 1961. However, to his dismay due to a slight discrepancy in his initial programme, the programme produced wildly divergent patterns. How was this possible? From an orderly linear framework, small differences in initial conditions should only lead to small differences in outcomes. But, in Lorenz's program, small discrepancies experienced feedback and reinforced themselves in chaotic ways producing radically divergent outcomes. Lorenz called this, the phenomenon where small changes in initial conditions lead to radically divergent outcomes in the same system, the 'butterfly effect', arguing that given the appropriate circumstances a butterfly flapping its wings in China could eventually lead to a tornado in the USA. Cause did not lead to effect. Order was not certain. Chaos/complexity was an integral part of physical phenomena. Moreover, phenomena could not be reduced and isolated, but should be seen as part of larger systems.

Other examples of complex systems can be found in simple forms of fluid dynamics. For example, the water molecules creating a vortex in your bathtub are a type of abiotic complex system. The molecules self-organise and form a stable complex system so long as the water lasts in the bathtub. The vortex is easy to recreate, but the exact combination of water molecules that made the specific vortex would be virtually impossible to recreate. Each vortex, though similar, is not an exact copy of the other. Another case is the movement of heated fluid in a contained space. As the fluid is heated it begins to organise itself into cylindrical rolls, heated fluid rising on one side and cooling on the other (the process of convection). However, when more heat is added, instability ensues and a wobble develops on the rolls. Add even more heat and the flow becomes wild and turbulent (Gleick 1988: 25).

One of the most famous and simple examples of this type of fluid-based complex system is the Lorenzian Waterwheel. This is a wheel that pivots around a centre point and has hanging buckets at the wheel's rim. The buckets have holes in the bottom. Water is poured in from the top. If the flow of water is too low, the bucket will not fill, friction will not be overcome and the wheel will not move. Increase the flow, the buckets will fill and the wheel will spin in one direction or another. However, increase the flow to a certain point and the buckets will not have time to empty on their upward journey. This will cause the spin to slow down and even reverse at chaotic intervals. In this way, even a simple linear mechanical system can exhibit chaotic non-linear behaviour.

This systems approach led to the creation of a variety of definitions of complex systems. In the abiotic world these systems are described as being *complex*, because they have numerous internal elements, *dynamic*, because their global behaviour is governed by local interactions between the elements, and *dissipative*, because they have to consume energy to maintain stable global patterns. Abiotic complex systems obey fundamental physical laws, but not in the same way as orderly linear systems. For example, the second law of thermodynamics, the most fundamental law of nature, states that when a system is left alone it drifts steadily into disorder. The effects of the second law are plain to see. A deserted building, for instance, eventually turns into a pile of rubble. After a few centuries even the rubble disappears without a trace. Ultimately, a system cut off from the outside world will fall into a deathly state of equilibrium in which change does not occur. For the complexity physicist Peter Allen, orderly equilibrium systems are 'dead' systems (Allen 2001).

Orderly linear systems are found at or near equilibrium. A ball bearing inside a bowl is a classic example; it quickly settles at the bottom and that is that. These systems can be very complicated. A jet engine is a wonderfully complicated piece of orderly machinery creating highly predictable physical outcomes that millions of pilots and passengers successfully depend upon every year. Complexity, by contrast, is exhibited by systems that are far from equilibrium. In this instance, the system has to exchange (dissipate) energy, or matter, with other systems in order to acquire and maintain self-organised stable patterns. That is the only option open to it to avoid falling into the destructive clutches of the second law of thermodynamics. The most dramatic illustration of that process is planet Earth. Without the nourishing rays of energy from the Sun, Earth would perish into complete equilibrium, and therefore nothingness. A continuous supply of energy from the Sun keeps the planet in a highly active state far from equilibrium. The energy is absorbed, dissipated and used to drive numerous local interactions that in total produce the stable pattern that we perceive as life on Earth.[3]

Visualising the range of abiotic phenomena can be done as shown in Figure 3.3 and Box 3.1.

Box 3.1 Golden rules for abiotic systems in a complexity paradigm

- **Partial order:** phenomena can exhibit both orderly and chaotic behaviours.
- **Reductionism and holism:** some phenomena are reducible, others are not.
- **Predictability and uncertainty:** phenomena can be partially modelled, predicted and controlled.
- **Probabilistic:** there are general boundaries to most phenomena, but within these boundaries exact outcomes are uncertain.

Complex systems in the biotic world

By the later half of the 20th century, with complexity already deeply penetrating the physical sciences, biologists, geneticists, environmentalists and physiologists also began to consider their respective disciplines within the

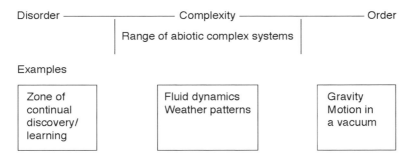

Figure 3.3 The range of abiotic phenomena in a complexity paradigm.

context of complexity. Analysts in these fields set out to investigate the properties of systems, including human beings, comprised of a large number of internal parts that interacted locally in what looked like a state of anarchy that somehow managed to engender self-organised, stable and sustainable global order. These systems were not only complex, dynamic and dissipative, but also adaptive and displayed *emergent properties* or *emergence*.

In the words of Murray Gell-Man, a Nobel prize-winning physicist, 'turbulent flow in a liquid is a complex system … But it doesn't produce a schema, a compression of information with which it can predict the environment' (Lewin 1999: 15). Without that schema, non-biological systems cannot respond to their environments in anything other than orderly, disorderly or abiotically complex ways. The ability of biotic complex systems to adapt and evolve creates a whole new range of complex outcomes. Likewise, biological complex systems are able to develop new emergent properties that may reshape the complex system as a whole and/or the subunits that make up the system. As Coveney and Highfield argue: 'Life is also an emergent property, one that arises when physiochemical systems are organized and interact in certain ways' (Coveney and Highfield 1995: 330).

From this perspective a whole new range of biotic complex systems began to be studied. For example, Kauffman was one of the first to view the genetic code as an evolving complex system (Kauffman 1993). Other concepts like autopoiesis, symbiosis and the *Gaia* system emerged to challenge the orderly framework in the biological sphere (Lovelock 1979; Dreamer and Fleischaker 1992; Capra 1996; Sole and Goodwin 2001). Due to the emergent nature of biological systems, the level of complexity can be significantly higher than those of abiotic phenomena and systems. Hence, on our simple scale of complexity, biotic complexity is placed on the more disorderly side of the scale than biotic complexity (*see* Figure 3.4 and Box 3.2).

Box 3.2 Golden rules for biotic systems in a complexity paradigm

- **Partial order:** phenomena can exhibit both orderly and chaotic behaviours.
- **Reductionism and holism:** some phenomena are reducible, others are not.

- **Predictability and uncertainty:** phenomena can be partially modelled, predicted and controlled.
- **Probabilistic:** there are general boundaries to most phenomena, but within these boundaries exact outcomes are uncertain.
- **Emergence:** they exhibit elements of adaptation and emergence.

A simple example of a biotic complex system would be the evolution of a species or the interaction of a given plant or animal in a particular ecosystem. A fish in a small pond will evolve and interact with the various food sources (small plants and animals) in the pond to create a stable complex system (such as a stable total number of fish). However, if a change is introduced to the system, a new competitor or food source, the fish may adapt and alter the nature of the system in totally unforeseen ways. Over time, new emergent properties may evolve in the system and/or in the fish itself.

A larger example is that of the concept of *Gaia*. As summarised in Coveney and Highfield (1995):

> *In 1968 James Lovelock upset gene-centered proponents of Darwin's views by arguing that the earth was not a ball of rock with a green layer of life on the surface. Biologists, following Darwin, see life adapting to its environment. The independently minded Lovelock viewed life and the environment as part of one superorganism in which creatures, rocks, air, and water interact in subtle ways to ensure that the environment remains stable ... feedback mechanisms are invoked to explain the relative constancy of the climate, the surprisingly moderate levels of salt in the oceans, the constant level of oxygen over the past few hundred million years, and why life forms are so diverse. Like it or hate it, simply looking for Gaia can give new insights into the complex feedback systems that rule the planet* (Coveney and Highfield 1995: 234–5).

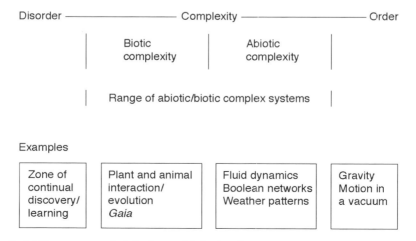

Figure 3.4 The range of abiotic and biotic phenomena.

Orderly (modernist) and disorderly (post-modernist) social science

The success of the orderly linear paradigm in the natural sciences had a profound effect on attitudes and practices in all sectors of human activity, spreading well beyond the disciplines embraced by the original scientific discoveries. The social sciences were no exception. Surrounded by the technological marvels of the industrial revolution which were founded on a Newtonian vision of an orderly, clockwork universe driven by observable and immutable laws, it did not take much of an intellectual leap to apply the lessons of the physical sciences to the social realm. The English philosopher Thomas Hobbes (1588–1678) used Newton's mechanistic vision to shape an orderly society, a *Leviathan*, that would save it from chaos and civil war. The French economist Francois Quesnay (1694–1774) and the *physiocrates* modelled the economic system on a mechanical clock. The French mathematician, philosopher and revolutionary politician, Condorcet (1743–1794) wrote while imprisoned by the Committee of Public Safety:

> *The sole foundation for belief in the natural sciences is the idea that the general laws directing the phenomena of the universe, known or unknown, are necessary and constant. Why should this principle be any less true for the development of the intellectual and moral faculties of man than for other operations of nature?* (Wilson 1999: 21).

The famous British economist Adam Smith (1723–1790) claimed to have captured the laws of economic interaction while his follower, David Ricardo (1772–1823) believed that some economic laws were 'as certain as the principles of gravitation' (Mainzer 1997: 264). Karl Marx (1818–1883) wedded his vision of class struggle to an analysis of the capitalist mode of production to create the 'immutable' and deterministic laws of capitalist development. Academics in all the major fields of social science welcomed the new age of certainty and predictability with open arms. Economics, politics, sociology all became 'sciences', desperate to duplicate the success of the natural sciences. Moreover, this desire was institutionalised through the development of modern universities that created and reinforced the disciplinarisation and professionalisation of the social sciences (Gulbenkian Commission 1996).

The high point of the linear paradigm was reached in the 1950s and 60s, particularly in universities in the United States. Strengthened by the success of planning programmes during the Second World War (WWII) and the early post-war period, pressured by the growing Cold War, and lavishly funded by the expanding universities, American academics strived to demonstrate, and hence control, the presumed rational nature of human interaction. This traditional Newtonian approach was clearly expressed in the modernisation theories of the Third World development, the realist vision of international relations, the behaviouralist writings of sociologists, the positivist foundations of liberal economics and the rational plans of public policy experts and urban planners.

Using the Newtonian frame of reference, modern social scientists unjustifiably assumed that physical and social phenomena were primarily linear and therefore predictable. They, consequently, applied reductionist methods founded on the belief that stable relationships exist between causes and effects, such as the assumption that individual self-interest is an explanation and/or a model for national level self-interest. Furthermore, based on this linear thinking they assumed that society and social institutions had an 'end-state' towards which they were evolving. Hence, economic interaction, democracy, fundamental social orders (communism, capitalism, development), etc all had final stages towards which they were evolving. Nation-states, societies and even individuals could be positioned along this developmental pathway, and policies could be devised to help them towards the next level.

The cultural embodiments of the orderly paradigm evolved in a variety of forms, ranging from Sherlock Holmes to Star Trek. Like a good linear social scientist, Holmes' 'scientific' study of crime enables him to solve all cases and astound his observers. As Holmes tries to make clear to Watson, there is nothing special about his powers, they are just a matter of method and effort. A similar belief in human rational capabilities underlies Star Trek's philosophy of 'to boldly go where no man has gone before'. In one episode from the 1960s series after the crew of the Enterprise have solved a local planetary difficulty, one crew member was concerned that the planet would revert to its former violent ways. The captain calmly responds that some 'sociologists' will be sent down to the planet to make sure that the problems won't happen again. The parallels to US 'advisors' in Vietnam or International Monetary Fund (IMF)/World Bank advisors in the Third World are all too obvious.

The remarkable dominance of the Newtonian frame of reference is brilliantly captured by a quotation from an early critic of the 'scientific' approach in politics argued in 1962:

> So deep and widespread is the belief, so eminent and able the believers in the value of the contemporary scientific study of politics, that there is not a little impatience with any attempt to question it ... All of us who profess the study of politics are confronted with the prevailing scientific approach, no matter how practical our concern, how slight our interest in methodology, or how keen our desire to get on with the business of direct investigation (Strong 1962: v).

The notable international success of Francis Fukuyama's book, *The End of History and the Last Man* (1993),[4] which claimed that history had reached its endpoint, demonstrated the continued influence of the linear framework. As Box 3.3 and Figure 3.5 summarise, orderly social science rests on the same foundation as orderly natural science, treated human beings like orderly atomistic objects and drew similar orderly conclusions.

Box 3.3   The foundations of orderly (modernist) social science

Theoretical basis
- Order
- Reductionism
- Predictability
- Determinism

Ontological/epistemological expectations
- Over time as human knowledge increases, phenomena will shift from the disorderly to the orderly side. *Social scientists are able to understand more and more about society and humanity.*
- Knowledge equals order. Hence, greater knowledge equals greater order. *Thus, history is progressive, leading to greater order.*
- With greater knowledge humans can increasingly predict and control more and more phenomena. *Those with greater knowledge can know more and thus should be in control.*
- There is an endpoint to phenomena and hence knowledge. *Once this endpoint is reached history stops and societal change comes to an end.*
- There is a hierarchy of scientific knowledge and methods with the orderly natural sciences at the zenith. Duplicating this knowledge and methods is the justification of orderly social science.

Methodological implications
- Researchers look for rational foundations to all phenomena.
- There are no inherent limits to human knowledge. The only constraints are effort and technology.
- Researchers can obtain predictable and repeatable experimental results.
- Duplicating orderly natural science methods is the primary methodological strategy.
- The creation of universal and parsimonious social laws is the ultimate goal.

However, even at its peak, countervailing tendencies in the social sciences survived. There is nothing new about questioning the fundamental order and rationality of human existence. Debates over these issues are easily traced back to Plato and Aristotle. A belief in the fundamentally rational and orderly nature of human existence only emerged in the Western philosophical tradition in the 17th and 18th centuries. Before this period, much of the human and physical world embraced unknowable mysteries that were cloaked in the enigmas of religion. During the 18th, 19th and 20th centuries, there continued to be a huge variety of potent critics of the mechanistic view and nature and society and of the limits of human rationality. In the late 18th century, the German scientist and philosopher, Immanuel Kant (1724–1804) argued

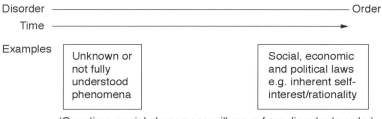

Figure 3.5 Range of outcomes for the paradigm of order.

that an organism 'cannot only be a machine, because a machine has only moving force; but an organism has an organising force ... which cannot be explained by mechanical motion alone' (Mainzer 1997: 83). These arguments plus the work of Friedrich Schelling (1775–1854) who described an organic 'science of living', and the writings of Goethe (1749–1832) who saw the mechanistic model of nature as 'grey ... like death ... a ghost and without sun' (Mainzer 1997: 84) created the foundation of the German romantic philosophy of nature which rejected the mechanism of Newton. In the early 20th century, the hermeneutical tradition of Sigmund Freud (1865–1939) and Max Weber (1864–1920) challenged the belief in the human rational capabilities and the degree to which humans can understand and control their environment and societies. In the mid-20th century, the American philosopher John Dewey (1859–1952) was espousing his philosophy of pragmatism as a strategy for dealing with the limits of knowledge and uniqueness of human experience. In the 1960s the famous Austrian economist FA Hayek argued that: 'in the field of complex phenomena the term "law" as well as the concepts of cause and effect are not applicable' (Hayek 1967: 42). By the 1970s, the influential French post-modernist philosopher Jean-Francois Lyotard, in *The Postmodern Condition: a report on knowledge,* was arguing for an end to all 'grand narratives' of Western society. Consequently, from the 1970s onwards as social scientists continually failed to capture the 'laws'[5] of society and economic interaction, and were continually frustrated over their inability to do so, they began to significantly question the Newtonian framework that underpinned political thinking on the left and right.

Out of this emerged the extremely diverse but significant challenge of (disorderly) post-modern position in social science. As defined by Terry Eagleton:

> *Postmodernism ... is a style of thought which is suspicious of classical notions of truth, reason, identity and objectivity, of the idea of universal progress or emancipation, of single frameworks, grand narratives or ultimate grounds of explanation. Against these Enlightenment norms, it sees the world as contingent, ungrounded, diverse, unstable, indeterminate, a set of disunified cultures or interpretations which breed a degree of scepticism about the objectivity of truth, history and norms, the givenness of natures and the coherence of identities* (Eagleton 1996: vii).

As excellently summarised by Colin Hay (2002), the post-modernist position stands in direct contrast to the traditional orderly (modernist) social science position. As we shall see, this drove post-modernists towards a strong 'anti-naturalist' (opposed to linking the natural and social sciences) position, seeing the study of society and humans as something entirely distinct from the study of nature and the physical world (*see* Box 3.4).

Box 3.4   The foundations of disorderly (post-modern) social science[a]

Ontological position
- The world is relational and experienced differently.
- Such experiences are culturally and temporally specific.
- Such experiences are singular and unique.
- They are neither linked by, nor expression of, generic processes.

Epistemological position (radical scepticism)
- Different subject positions inform different knowledge claims.
- Knowledge is perspectival and different perspectives are incommensurate.
- Truth claims cannot be adjudicated empirically.
- The assertion of truth claims are dogmatic and potentially totalitarian.

Methodological position (deconstruction):
- undermines strong knowledge claims
- undermines modernist assumption of a privileged access to reality that is untenable and potentially totalitarian in its effects
- uses deconstructivist techniques to disrupt modernist meta-narratives, drawing attention to otherwise marginalised 'others'.

Range of outcomes for the post-modernist paradigm of contested order (disorder)
- Multiple contested relational 'orders' which rise and fall over time, but have no developmental path or direction.

[a]This information is adapted from Hay 2002: 227.

It is important to note that post-modernism, by its own disorderly nature, has never been as structured and coherent as the modernist paradigm. Moreover, post-modernists' anti-naturalist tendencies have generally kept them at arm's-length from the natural and physical sciences. Hence, the post-modernist critique has mainly occurred within the social sciences. Despite these limitations it has had a profound impact on the social sciences, forcing many in such diverse fields as international relations, political science and sociology to address its fundamentally disorderly and irrationalist arguments. In general, however, other fields, particularly economics, have held on tightly to the linear Newtonian framework, while others drifted towards a middling position between the extremes of a strictly scientific Newtonian framework and the fundamentally irrationalist reflectivist one.[6] It is this division and debate that has led the social sciences to the threshold of a 'scientific revolution' that could shift them into a complexity paradigm.

Complexity and social science

The next question to ask is, how do human beings fit into the complexity paradigm? They are an obvious symbiotic part of the complex web of their physical and biological surroundings. Nevertheless, what makes them distinct from this environment? Their most fundamental difference is consciousness: the ability to ask 'Who am I?', 'How did I get here?', 'What does life mean?'. This ability to be self-aware, to understand aspects of the world around them, be aware of their history and to evolve interpretations of themselves, their surroundings and their history makes human beings fundamentally different from all other life forms and physical phenomena. However, this interpretive ability does not produce orderly interpretations. The uniqueness of individual human experience combined with multitudinous possibilities of collective human interaction and the evolutionary nature of human society produce a very high degree of complex interpretive outcomes. Therefore, conscious interpretive outcomes (norms, values, historical interpretation) must be positioned on the more disorderly side of our complexity scale. This does not imply that there are no universal norms, values or interpretations. For example, a prohibition against murder is a common societal trait. However, the definition of murder, the mitigating circumstances that could surround it and the punishment for the act all vary widely over time and between different societies and cultures. The position of conscious phenomena is outlined in Figure 3.6 and Box 3.5.

Box 3.5 Golden rules of conscious systems in a complexity paradigm

- **Partial order:** phenomena can exhibit both orderly and chaotic behaviours.
- **Reductionism and holism:** some phenomena are reducible, others are not.
- **Predictability and uncertainty:** phenomena can be partially modelled, predicted and controlled.
- **Probabilistic:** there are general boundaries to most phenomena, but within these boundaries exact outcomes are uncertain.
- **Emergence:** they exhibit elements of adaptation and emergence.
- **Interpretation:** the actors in the system can be aware of themselves, the system and their history and may strive to interpret and direct themselves and the system.

Complexity theory does not disprove the rationalist paradigm or its antithesis (post-modernism), but acts like a synthesis or bridge between the naturalism of rationalism and the anti-naturalism of post-modernism and creates a new framework which bridges the two opposing positions. Both orderly modernism and disorderly post-modernism are equally flawed. Both assume that humanity and its relationship to the natural are inherently orderly or disorderly when in reality they are both. This bridging position is summarised in Table 3.1.

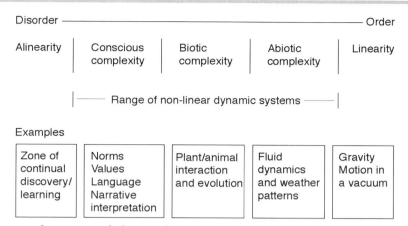

Figure 3.6 The range of abiotic, biotic and conscious phenomena.

Table 3.1 Summary of fundamental positions of modern, complexity and post-modern science

Modern	Complexity	Post-modern
Epistemological position		
Order	Partial order	Relational
Rationality	Bounded rationality	Relational rationality
Predictability	Predictability and uncertainty	Unpredictable
Reductionism	Reductionism and holism	Irreducible
Determinism	Probabilistic and emergent	Indeterminate
Non-interpretive	Interpretive	Relational interpretation
Relation of physical and social sciences		
Subservient/inferiority relationship. Social science must strive to duplicate methods and results of physical science	Integrative relationship. No necessary separation between physical and social sciences	No clear relationship exists. Relational and interpretative nature of humanity makes clear relationship difficult
Relation of humanity to nature		
Expanding human dominance over nature	Holistic interpretation of human and natural symbiotic co-evolution	Unclear relational distinction between humans and nature
Methodological implications		
Experimentation, quantification and search for fundamental laws	Integration of experimentation and interpretation; fundamental laws and distinctive outcomes	Relational interpretations and undermining truth claims

Table 3.1 Summary of fundamental positions of modern, complexity and post-modern science (continued)

Modern	Complexity	Post-modern
Vision of progress		
There are no inherent limits to human knowledge and progress	There are significant limits to knowledge and progress due to complexity and uncertainty	No fundamental order. Pure knowledge creation and progress is impossible to know
History is progressive, cumulative, and leads to an ultimate end	History may progress and display fundamental patterns, but it is also uncertain and tortuous	History is relational hence it does not universally progress

More importantly, for the social sciences if one accepts a complexity framework then one must abandon the rigid divisions and certainties of both modern and post-modern science and recognise the integrative nature of the physical and social sciences. Complexity theory argues that physical and social reality is composed of a wide range of interacting orderly, complex and disorderly phenomena. One can focus on different aspects, orderly (gravity or basic aspects of existence: life/death), complex (species evolution or institutional development) or disorderly (random chance or irrationality), but that does not mean that the others do not exist. Consequently, complexity theory demands a broad and open-minded approach to epistemological positions and methodological strategies without universalising particular positions or strategies. As Richardson and Cilliers argued:

> If we allow different methods, we should allow them without granting a higher status to some of them. Thus, we need both mathematical equations and narrative descriptions. Perhaps one is more appropriate than the other under certain circumstances, but one should not be seen as more scientific than the other (Richardson and Cilliers 2001: 12).

These conclusions 'bridge the old divide between the two worlds (of natural and human sciences) without privileging the one above the other' (Richardson and Cilliers 2001: 11).

A strategy for conceptualising the integrative nature of complexity is to look at how all types of complexity dynamics are reflected in the human condition. For example, using Figure 3.7 as a template we can produce an overview of the range of complexity dynamics of human phenomena. The key point to recognise is that there are both orderly and disorderly dynamics and that they are not hierarchically organised. A given human outcome, a decision to have coffee at breakfast or bomb a particular village, could be based on orderly, complex and disorderly dynamics with all being equally essential to the final outcome.

Beginning with linearity, the most fundamental and universalistic elements of human complexity are basic physiological functioning, in particular life and

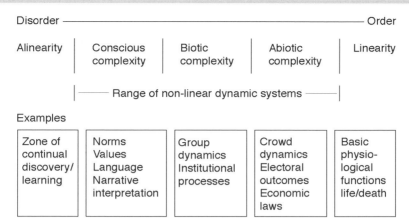

Figure 3.7 **The range of complexity dynamics in human phenomena.**

death. These physical boundaries and requirements, carbon-based life forms requiring air, water and food to survive and reproduce, are the most orderly aspects of human existence. Deprived of these fundamentals, a human will die. What could be more orderly?

Moving into the range of complex systems, examples of mechanistic complexity in human systems would involve situations where individuals were forced to act in a mechanistic fashion. Traffic dynamics, choosing one road or another, crowd dynamics, choosing one exit or another, and electoral outcomes, choosing one candidate or another, are all examples of mechanical complex systems. Like mechanical complex systems, relatively simple and stable patterns will emerge. However, this is no guarantee that these patterns will be continuously stable (traffic jams, crowd delays, landslide elections), nor is it possible to perfectly recreate the exact conditions of these events at a later time. The golden rules of abiotic complex systems apply.

Examples of organic complex systems in the human world can easily be seen in the organisational dynamics of economic and social institutions. As demonstrated by the huge growth in management and complexity literature, a business is a complex system that interacts with a larger complex environment (the market) that is very similar to the earlier model of a fish in a pond. General patterns emerge and the business is able to adapt to changes in its environment, but exact predictions and explanations of how a change in the environment will affect the business, or the best strategies for the business to survive in the altered environment are impossible to know in advance.

An added layer of complexity in the human condition is its faculty of consciousness. Human beings create signs, symbols, myths, narratives and discourse in order to understand, control and exchange information about their surroundings. This ability adds another layer of complexity onto the human condition that is distinctive from the natural world. Examples of this conscious complexity include the creation of language, norms and values and discourse, and can be taken from virtually any type of human verbal interaction. A seemingly simple student–teacher relationship can be layered in historically, culturally and personally specific aspects that would be impossible to recreate in a different time and place.

Lastly, like the natural world, alinear human phenomena are nearly impossible to explain using examples since they are without a pattern and would have to be completely random. The closest common human experiences that readily come to mind would be the chaotic nature of dreams and the unconscious, random effects of certain disorders on the complex functioning of the brain and the phenomena of luck.

How can all of these dynamics be combined to explain human phenomena? Let us begin with the phenomenon of going to a shop to get a cup of coffee. I have a basic human need for water and nutrition that is very orderly and highly predictable. This is combined in the case of the coffee with the desire for a mildly addictive stimulant. As I leave my home to walk to the coffee shop, I immediately encounter crowd dynamics that may speed or impede my progress to the shops. When I reach my favourite coffee shop, I see that a new coffee shop is open on the opposite corner of the street, competing for my business. These shops are engaged in the complex biotic process of competition. In a process of conscious complexity, I am enticed to enter the new shop by its pleasant name, 'Vic's Coffee Shop', which reminds me of my childhood. As I enter the shop a woman is leaving with a cup of coffee. I open the door for her and say 'good morning'. As she turns to thank me a fly randomly lands on her face, blown there by a turbulent gust of wind from a passing bus. She has a dreadful fear of insects from the stories her grandmother used to tell her as a child, and immediately flinches from the touch of the fly. The coffee spills, mostly on my pants. I return, change my pants and make a cup of coffee for myself at home. The point of detailing my pursuit of coffee is to demonstrate the remarkable linear, complex and alinear processes that are the foundation of most commonplace events in human existence.

But what if the stakes are higher, when lives are at stake? Does complexity still apply? In 1971 Graham Allison, a leading Professor of Political Science at Harvard University, wrote *The Essence of Decision*, one of the greatest English language books in international relations and the best book on the Cuban missile crisis. The basic story is well known. In 1962, responding to the deployment of US nuclear missiles in Turkey, the USSR began secretly deploying missile bases in Cuba. The bases were discovered and a blockade imposed on Cuba. The USSR challenged the blockade and threatened nuclear war, but eventually backed down, dismantling the bases in Cuba. On the surface this would seem to be a simple game of threat and counter-threat that luckily for the lives of hundreds of millions did not go wrong. At one level this is correct. On the other hand, as Allison brilliantly demonstrated, several different political and bureaucratic dynamics both between and within the USSR and USA were going on at the same time. Seemingly rational and irrational strategies emerge from the interplay of these dynamics. For example, when the Soviets were building the missile bases, they built them out in the open and in the same pattern as their bases in the USSR, making them easy to detect by US spyplanes, a clear strategic blunder. This was not caused by military stupidity or poor implementation, but by the centralised control over Soviet military engineers. The engineers were told to build missile bases in Cuba. They had a model from the USSR, in the open and in a certain pattern, and they did as they were told. On the US side, the decision to form a naval blockade to stop the Soviets shipping the missiles to Cuba was fraught with military, bureaucratic and personal rivalries. In the end it may have come down to President Kennedy's personal naval experience that led him to choose a naval option. Overall, as Allison points out, these different dynamics could explain parts of the crisis, but none explained all of it. As President John F Kennedy said after the crisis:

> *The essence of ultimate decision remains impenetrable to the observer – often, indeed, to the decider himself ... There will always be the dark and tangled stretches in the decision-making process – mysterious even to those who may be most intimately involved* (Allison 1971: vi).

Debates in complexity science

Not surprisingly, due to its growing popularity, evolution as a 'New Age selling feature' (Thrift 1999) and, most importantly, the breadth of its macro- and meta-theoretical implications, complexity theory generates a significant variation in theoretical interpretations.[7] Detailing these differences is clearly beyond the boundaries of this chapter. However, understanding the difference between modernist and post-modernist interpretations of complexity is important since it will have direct relevance to later applications.

For some, complexity is a strategy for going beyond a linear paradigm, but maintaining a modernist and progressive vision. In one of the major books on complexity and the social sciences, David Byrne, claiming to follow in the footsteps of the scientific realism of the philosopher Roy Bhaskar (Bhaskar 1986), argued that while 'positivism was dead ... and starting to smell' (Byrne 1998: 37) and the relativism of post-modernism was 'bone idleness promoted to a meta-theoretical programme' (Byrne 1998: 45):

> *complexity/chaos offers the possibility of an engaged science not founded in pride, in the assertion of an absolute knowledge as the basis for social programmes, but rather in a humility about the complexity of the world coupled with a hopeful belief in the potential of human beings for doing something about it* (Byrne 1998: 45).

Moreover, for Byrne:

> *complexity accounts are foundationalist* [can provide a foundation for further knowledge], *although they are absolutely not reductionist and positivist ...* [and] *are surely part of the modernist programme* (Byrne 1998: 35).

For others, in particular Paul Cilliers, complexity is best understood by post-modernists, particularly those working in the tradition of Derrida and Lyotard, because their theories 'have an implicit sensitivity for the complexity of the phenomena they deal with'(Cilliers 1998: xii). Cilliers certainly agrees with Byrne that complexity is non-reductionist and anti-positivist, but stresses that:

> *Claiming that self-organisation is an important property of complex systems is to argue against foundationalism. The dynamic nature of self-organisation, where the structure of the system is continuously transformed through the*

interaction of contingent, external factors and historical, internal factors, cannot be explained by resorting to a single origin or to an immutable principle ... self-organisation provides the mechanism whereby complex structure can evolve without having to postulate first beginnings ... It is exactly in this sense that postmodern theory contributes to our understanding of complex self-organising systems (Cilliers 1998: 106).

Generally, both authors have much in common. They both see the complexity framework as a challenge to linearity and reductionism. They both reject the relativism of some strands of post-modernism and argue that formal modelling is still possible, though significantly restrained under a complexity framework.

Their differences are primarily those of degree and allegiances to certain theoretical traditions, but are important. For Byrne, coming from a more modernist orientation, complex systems theory represents a type of progress. In essence, more phenomena can be understood, which enables individuals and state actors to exert more control over their lives and societies. For Cilliers, with a more post-modern orientation, complexity theory emphasises the uncertain and contingent, and thus may expand our understanding, but cannot constitute a foundation for pure knowledge and hence be a gauge for progress. These differences are due to the level of complexity theory that one concentrates on. At its meso-/macro-theoretical level, complexity theory provides new tools for understanding these systems, hence it does seem progressive. At the same time, at the meta-theoretical level, it stresses that there are always orderly, complex and disorderly phenomena. Although one may be able to develop new ways and systems for understanding orderly and complex phenomena, there is always uncertainty and contingency in complex phenomena, and the uncharted realm of disorder. Hence, it can appear as both foundationalist and anti-foundationalist.

Lastly, although neither Byrne nor Cilliers explicitly discuss it, complexity has obvious implications for both naturalists and anti-naturalists (those who support and oppose the use of physical science theories and methods in the social sciences). Again, drawing on critical realism and the 'non-positivist' or 'critical' naturalism of Bhaskar, both try to use complexity as a bridge to link the natural and social sciences. Both want to break down the barriers between the major fields of knowledge, mirroring the conclusions of the Gulbenkian Commission, but neither wants to impose a new unifying 'scientific' law on the social realm. In essence, they want to open up the sciences, 'not only towards the world, but also internally. The barriers between the various scientific disciplines need to be crossed' (Cilliers 1998: 127). In this sense, complexity theory is a direct challenge to strong naturalists and anti-naturalists who argue for the complete dominance or distinctiveness of one type of science over or from another, or who reject the possibility of some types of generalisable scientific knowledge.

A question of method

As mentioned above, complexity implies methodological pluralism. However, this does not mean that all methodological strategies are appropriate for all phenomena. Linear, reductionist, quantitative and predictive methods can be more applicable to certain social phenomena and less so to others. This goes for non-linear methods as well. An excellent way for visually conceptualising this constrained methodological pluralism was created by David Harvey and Michael Reed. Building on the work of Kenneth Boulding and Neil Smelser, they created a hierarchy of ontological complexity in social systems. By combining this on a matrix with a linear layout of levels of modelling abstraction, more linear (left) to less linear (right), they produced a table as shown in Table 3.2.

Table 3.2 The general range of fit between the level of complexity in social phenomena and the general range of methodological strategies (Kiel and Elliot 1997: 307)

Levels of complexity in social phenomena	Levels of modelling abstraction (from left to right, moving from more prediction to greater description)				
Alinear				X	X
Conscious complexity			X	X	X
Biotic complexity		X	X	X	
Abiotic complexity	X	X	X		
Linear	X	X			
	Predictive modelling	Statistical modelling	Ideal-type modelling	Historical narratives	Interpretive techniques

One could certainly quibble over the exact divisions of ontological complexity or whether more methods could be added to the left or right of the levels of modelling. Nevertheless, the underlying principle that only extremely orderly or disorderly phenomena can be explored with one or a few methodological strategies, while the vast range of complex social phenomena require a fuller panoply of methodological strategies, undermines hierarchical assumptions about methodologies and rejects a radical relativist position as well.

As briefly discussed in the introduction to this book, the case studies will rely heavily on institutional and historical narratives combined with comparative ideal-type modelling. This does not preclude more statistical and predictive modelling for the more linear aspects of the EU–UK welfare state relationship. In fact, many of complexity's most exciting discoveries and biggest claims come from its potential in the field of computer modelling. Detailed discussions and descriptions of these modelling techniques are readily available and are increasingly being explored by a growing range of social scientists.[8] However, it is beyond the range of this book and will have to be dealt with by others.

Complexity and the politics of order

Why is the complexity framework so radical and important? The Newtonian paradigm had much to commend it. It helped to lift the miasma of religious interpretation from the eyes of Renaissance thinkers. It fired the desire of countless academics, scientists and philosophers 'to strive, to seek, to find and not to yield',[9] and was the foundation of the industrial revolution. Its fundamental weakness was its arrogance. For a Newtonian thinker, with the complete knowledge of nature and humanity, they could be gods and create heaven on Earth. By the 20th century, flushed with the heady success of mechanistic and industrial achievement and the growing power and capabilities of the state, no problem seemed beyond the grasp of humanity. Social scientists merely wedded this orderly vision and arrogance to the social realm and produced the fundamental visions of social order, communism and capitalism, which structured the history of the 20th century. Many had the best of intentions, hoping to make the world of better place for all time, the final order. That these visions led to the extreme forms of human suffering and environmental degradation in large parts of the globe was certainly a setback for their dreams and the Newtonian framework.

In the EU–UK context, as we will argue later, much of the UK debate surrounding the EU and its policies is shaped by an implicit orderly Newtonian framework. Anti-Europeans are often complaining that the EU is too disorderly, messy and/or incoherent to function as a true state. This implies that there is a set form or endpoint that the EU must reach if it is ever to become legitimate. Interestingly, this is the same type of mental framework that shapes the thinking of pro-Europeans within the UK. For them, if the EU does not obtain certain powers or structures it will be left 'unfinished'. From a complexity perspective, the EU is an evolving process that has a stable fundamental framework but is open enough to allow for a vast range of distinctive local interactions and developments. The very messiness of the EU is one of its major hidden strengths.

Does this mean the end of progress? Are we back to Nietzschean nihilism or Heideggerian fatalism in the face of forces beyond our control? Complexity is clearly focused on attacking the cult of order. However, complexity is an equal challenge to the cult of disorder. That human beings cannot be gods, that we live in a symbiotic relationship with each other and nature, and that we do not have complete control over our lives and hence complete freedom does not imply failure and apathy. As a leading complexity thinker, Klaus Mainzer, put it:

> *The complex system approach cannot explain to us* what *life is. But it can show us* how *complex and sensitive life is. Thus it can help us to become aware of the value of our life* (Mainzer 1997: 325).

Reverting to apathy will not solve our problems and may easily lead our complex human system into a more negative 'attractor state'. The need to respond to the threat of global warming immediately springs to mind. In essence, apathy is just as blind as a desperate attempt to find the new, new order or to buttress and defend an existing one. The problem with both the orderist and disorderist positions is that they refuse to recognise the complex and uncertain reality that surrounds them. That it is uncertain does not mean it cannot progress, but it will not progress in a clear path. In some ways a disorderist position is as arrogant as an orderist position, both know the future. One is desperate to make the present squeeze into a given future. The other is unwilling to do anything about the present because it is already heading to a given future.

Once one abandons the arrogance of order and disorder and accepts the humbling limits of knowledge and uncertain potential which complexity implies, then a new politics emerges: a politics of uncertainty, but also of openness, of mistakes and learning, of failure and adaptation. Exploring this new politics in the context of the EU–UK relationship is what this book is all about. However, before we can begin this exploration, we need to explore how complexity theory relates to and reinterprets European integration and UK welfare state theory.

Notes

[1]   For a philosophical discussion of the process of transformation, including the switch from linear to non-linear thinking, *see* Fuller (1997). Hawkings (1988: 1–14), on the other hand, provides an insightful technical analysis of the way scientific beliefs and methods changed through the ages. The uncertainty principle advanced by Heisenberg had a particularly pivotal impact on the future course of scientific research. For a review of developments in physics *see* Barrow *et al.* (2004).

[2]   Major works on complexity include: Gleick (1988); Capra (1991); Kauffman (1993, 1995); Gell-Mann (1994); Coveney and Highfield (1995); Bar-Yam (1997); Waldrop (1992).

[3]   The literature on the complexity paradigm and abiotic complex systems has now become quite large. Key works include Nicolis and Prigogine (1989); Kauffman (1993, 1995); Coveney and Highfield (1992). In addition, Waldrop (1994) and Lewin (1999) present an excellent general introduction to complexity.

[4]   Fukuyama's 'End of history' thesis continues to resonate with elite and mass opinion particularly after the events of September 11. *See* Fukuyama's article 'How the West has won', *The Guardian,* 11 October 2001.

[5]   For a review of the role of laws in the social sciences *see* Martin and McIntyre (1994).

[6]   For discussions of the development of the debate between these two sides *see* Bhaskar (1986); Delanty (1997); Byrne (1998); Cilliers (1998); Bevir (1999); Rasch and Wolfe (2000).

[7]   Non-linear systems theory (complexity theory) has established footholds in all of the major areas of social science. In philosophy and social theory *see* Byrne (1998); Cilliers (1998). In economics *see* Barnett *et al.* (1989); Day and Samuelson (1994); Mirowski (1994); Ormerod (1994, 1998); Hodgson (1997). In organisational and management theory *see* Stacey (1999) and Stacey *et al.* (2000). In sociology and politics *see* Eve *et al.* (1997); Kiel and Elliot (1997); Cioffi-Revilla (1998); Rycroft and Kash (1999). In development theory *see* Rihani and Geyer (2001) and Rihani (2002). In political theory *see* Geyer (2003b) and Scott (1998). In international relations *see* Jervis (1997). For an excellent overview of the spread of complexity theory and a critical review of its popularisers *see* Thrift (1999).

[8]   Examples include: Krasner (1990); Axelrod (1997); Grebogi and Yorke (1997); Axelrod and Cohen (2000).

[9]   Tennyson *Ulysses* 1842: L.67.

Chapter 4

Using complexity to reinterpret the EU–UK social policy relationship

Before exploring our case studies, we need to take one more preliminary step. Having gone through the EU–UK social policy relationship, the problem of complexity and complexity theory, we must now focus on how complexity reinterprets the EU–UK social policy relationship. This we will do by examining how complexity casts new light on European integration and UK social policy in general, and then on the EU–UK social policy relationship in particular.

How does complexity theory reinterpret European integration?

As we saw in Chapter 2, international relations (IR) and European integration (EI) theory at the end of the 20th century had gone through remarkably similar changes. First, since the 1970s there has been a significant challenge to the hegemonic position of the rationalist paradigm in IR and EI theory. Second, linked to this challenge has been the growing recognition of human and social complexity. Third, a core division has emerged within the discipline between rationalists who adopt a strong naturalist position, modelling themselves on a traditional view of the natural sciences, and reflectivists who adopt an anti-naturalist position and oppose the use of natural science epistemologies and methods in the human sphere. Lastly, constructivists have attempted to bridge this division by emphasising the importance of broader ontologies, but have been rejected and/or co-opted by both sides.

How does complexity theory fit into these debates? Unsurprisingly, the growth of complexity in the social sciences has begun to spill over into IR and EU theory (Jervis 1997; Geyer 2003a; Rengger 2000). As we have seen, complexity theory argues that order, complexity and disorder all play a role in the creation of the natural and human world. For complexity theory, there are orderly, complex and disorderly phenomena and different epistemological and methodological strategies apply to each. Universal laws and order only apply to certain phenomena. This implies that the fundamental naturalist–anti-naturalist division within the IR and EI theory is based on an out-of-date view of the natural sciences. The natural sciences have not stood still. They have gone through a Kuhnian paradigmatic shift that challenges the traditional naturalist–anti-naturalist division (Kuhn 1970). Without this division, neither rationalists nor reflectivists can claim to have a superior grasp of reality or a greater access to the 'truth' since both are only describing part of the picture and 'the divisions between "rationalist" and "reflectivist" ... will become progressively harder to draw' (Rengger 2000: 195).

Can the international arena and European Union be interpreted as complex systems?

The easiest way to view the international arena as a complex system is to insert it into the complexity framework developed in Chapter 3 (*see* Figure 4.1).

The short-term basic framework of the system, particularly its significant power inequalities, appears as its most obvious linear aspects. Nation-states have been significant actors, have experienced power inequalities and struggled to adapt and change; these are all parts of what appears to be a basic framework of the international system. The power of the USA significantly influences its range of options for responding to events such as those of 11 September. However, dynamics similar to abiotic complexity can be immediately perceived within the procedures of the international institutions and regimes (United Nations (UN), regional and trade organisations, etc) that pervade the international system. The voting pattern in the UN of supporting the USA in its 'war on terrorism' led to a recognisable pattern of responses from various countries. However, the exact reasons behind these decisions or that an exact group would support a later 'war on terrorism' would be extremely hard to predict.

Dynamics similar to those found in biotic complex systems can easily be identified in the adaptive and interactive strategies that emerge when international institutions, states and non-state actors interact with each other. For example, as the USA began talking about expanding the 'war on terrorism' to include other nations (North Korea, Libya, etc), they upset the balance in the coalition which was supporting the actions in Afghanistan. Allies began to weaken their support and question other areas, such as Palestinian conflict in Israel, of US international policy. This was obviously complicated by the conscious complexity of competing norms and interpretations of the 'war' and US policies. A good example would be the different interpretations of the treatment and rights of the prisoners at Camp X-ray at Guantánamo Bay. Finally, the exact long-term development of the international system would seem to be the most uncertain and unpredictable analysis. How could an observer of the international system of 1900 have predicted the rise of communism, two world wars and the hegemony of the USA by 1950? How could an observer in 1950 have predicted the economic success of the West, collapse of communism and rise of the European

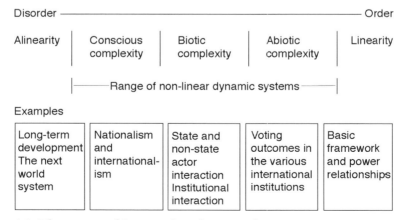

Figure 4.1 The range of international arena phenomena.

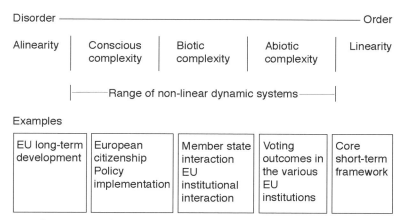

Figure 4.2 The range of European Union phenomena.

Union by 2000? The range of possible developments and interactions is enormously large.

In a similar fashion the EU can easily be inserted into a complexity framework (*see* Figure 4.2).

The most linear aspect of the EU is its core short-term framework. There is a very high degree of probability (near linearity) that the basic structures of the EU (core member state voting balances, institutional structures, power relationships) will remain stable in the short term. The various voting procedures in the EU Parliament and Council demonstrate aspects of abiotic complexity of the EU. Choices are constrained by having to vote for or against a particular proposal, and may produce stable patterns (certain member states or groups always voting for/against certain proposals). However, the pattern is not continuously stable, nor can one be certain that similar voting patterns at different times were based on the exact same factors. For example, the Scandinavian countries may generally vote as a block on most proposals, demonstrating a stable pattern, but their exact reasons for doing so may vary substantially with every proposal.

As any multilevel governance theorist would point out, aspects of biotic complexity are most obvious in the multiple types of member state and EU institutional interaction. Member states and EU institutions are constantly interacting in evolving and adaptive ways to new policies and developments within the EU system. Stable patterns emerge, but these are much more susceptible to unpredictable developments as different member states and institutions constantly evolve and adjust to new opportunities and constraints. For example, many observers of EU social policy expected it to expand rapidly after the defeat of the British Conservative Government in 1997. However, despite a more receptive pro-social policy Labour Government other supposedly pro-EU social policy member states suddenly became less supportive. The basic pattern of limited EU social policy developments continued, but the internal dynamics were transformed (Geyer 2000a).

Conscious complexity is most obvious in areas such as the meaning of EU citizenship and the implementation of EU policies in the member states. EU citizenship is an extremely contested concept and means drastically different things to the various member states and groups within the member states. This is complicated by the continual evolution of the norms surrounding 'citizenship' within the member states themselves and how the actions of the EU, its policies, are implemented and interpreted by the member states and their populations.

A good example of the alinear nature of the EU would be assumptions of its long-term development. There are so many possible outcomes of the mechanical, organic and conscious complex systems with and surrounding the EU, that predicting its exact development in the long term is obviously an alinear exercise. Again, imagine the response of the average European in 1950 if you were told that in little over 50 years' time the European Coal and Steel Community will have 25 members, comprise the largest economic unit in the world and have powers in virtually every major policy area. You would be immediately identified as slightly cracked or a complete Euro-lunatic. At best, one can guess or pick a future that one would like to see, but it will have virtually no direct relationship to the one that will emerge. This does not mean that it will have no relationship to the future. The 'dreams' of the pro-Europeans certainly cast a long shadow over its current reality, just not in the way they would have expected.

General implications

If the EU and international system can be interpreted as complex systems, then there are several major implications. First, this implies 'incompressibility', that any truly accurate description must be as complex as the system itself. Hence, the pursuit of parsimonious order must of necessity take the observer further and further from holistic reality. Second, since the EU and international systems are composed of different phenomena then one must accept methodological pluralism; quantitative modelling, qualitative analysis, historical description and narrative discourse all have their place with regard to particular phenomena. There is no universal hierarchy of phenomena and hence no hierarchy of method. Third, this uncertainty or perceived lack of knowledge is actually a strength of human systems since:

> *it is this very 'ignorance' or multiple misunderstandings that generates microdiversity, and leads therefore to exploration and (imperfect) learning* (Allen 2001: 41).

This means that different interpretations, diverse interests, uncertain responses, clumsy adaptations, learning and mistakes are what keep a system healthy and evolving. Truly orderly systems, where all of the elements are at the average or are in agreement, are dead systems and have no ability to explore new patterns or adapt to new environments.

The EU itself provides an excellent example of the healthy nature of complexity. From an orderly rationalist framework it is incomprehensively messy. From a reflectivist standpoint it cannot possibly order the multifaceted and multilevel nature of its constituent societies and subgroups. Nevertheless, it exists and thrives as an excellent set of institutions for promoting complex interaction, learning, diversity and adaptation at the subnational, national and European levels. Just imagine how long the EU would last if it did try to assert a comprehensive rigid order on the multitude of member states. Even its most rigid policies, such as European Monetary Union (EMU), allow for a surprising amount of hidden flexibility and adaptation. In fact, it is the very flexibility of the other aspects of economic policy that allows the member states to accept the rigidity within the European monetary order. As Hodson and Maher explain in relation to the EU's 'open method of coordination' (developed for the 2000 Lisbon European Council) for promoting economic and social policy cooperation:

> This is no formal attempt to control outcomes (outside of fiscal policy of course), and process is determined by a system of benchmarking and lesson-drawing, emphasizing state competence and the voluntary alignment of policies ... The desire of the EC to control outcomes, as manifest in the directive as the rule of choice in the single market, with its emphasis on common outcomes if not methods, is overcome by recognition of the importance of diversity at the national level in relation to policy formation, legal frameworks, ideational references and popular perceptions and reactions to either the European project generally or the specific policy being co-ordinated (Hodson and Maher 2001: 731).

In essence, European integration is not a threat because it combines an agreed fundamental framework with member state diversity and autonomy. This was not based on any pre-ordained plan, but emerged from a multifaceted combination of historical events and political economic structures including the weakness of the EU as a power centre, the continuing resilience of the member states to oppose centralising EU initiatives and the evolving nature of the international system. A significant change in any of these factors could easily have disrupted the seemingly reasonable complex development of European integration and Europeanisation.

How does complexity theory reinterpret UK social policy?

As discussed in Chapter 2, one of the most influential recent theories of the UK welfare state and social policy is the concept of Anthony Giddens' 'third way'. The foundation of the third way rests on Giddens' interpretation of manufactured risk/uncertainty, the nature of social reflexivity, the desire to 'go beyond left and right' and his longing to be radical. For Giddens, as human actions have increasingly come to dominate the natural world and humans have increasingly replaced external orderly risks with human-manufactured disorderly risks (global warming, nuclear devastation, etc), the interface between humans and nature has become increasingly complex. This new manufactured uncertainty is further complicated by the increasing social reflexivity of individuals in the post-modern world. Not only do they have to confront manufactured uncertainty, but they are no longer willing to believe in or submit to traditional authorities or ideologies. Hence, traditional ideologies of left and right are increasingly outdated and useless in the current age.

On all of these aspects, complexity theory would agree, but go a step further. Yes, traditional ideologies are outdated, manufactured risks have increased and individuals have become more socially reflexive. However, complexity theory would stress that the natural world and external risks were never completely orderly. In fact they have always been complex interaction between humans and nature with unpredictable consequences. Human interaction with the weather and plants and animals, to take just two obvious examples, has led to a multitude of complex outcomes throughout the history of humanity, from the plague to the potato famine. Consequently, there has always been a degree of manufactured risk, and humans have attempted to deal with it in similar ways. Even in pre-modern societies, human beings attempted to deal with manufactured risks by promoting strategies of social order. Countertendencies to these strategies emerged and even reconciling 'third ways'.[1] Thus, when critics of the third way complain that it is 'nothing new', they are more correct than they know.

What is unique about the Newtonian linear framework of the 18th, 19th and 20th centuries was the degree to which humans believed that they could order their societies. Flushed with the heady success of mechanistic and industrial achievement, no problem seemed beyond the grasp of humanity. Social scientists merely wedded this vision to the social realm and produced the fundamental visions of social order, communism and capitalism, which structured the history of the 20th century. From a complexity perspective, both visions of order were never possible. Full-blown communism where the state dominated every economic transaction, and full-blown capitalism where the market determined all social interactions were equally unsustainable within the complex interaction between humans and nature. Generally, it was the pursuit of these extreme forms of order which brought about extreme forms of human suffering: the repression, death and suffering that the Soviet peoples experienced, particularly during the 1930s, is mirrored in the repression, death and suffering brought on the Third World by World Bank/International Monetary Fund (IMF) structural adjustment programmes implementing extreme forms of marketisation on their societies.

At first glance, Giddens' third way seems to pursue a similar strategy regarding left and right. He is critical of both market and state extremes and produces a raft of policies and proposals that blend elements of both. However, he also wants to recapture, for the left, the 'future-oriented radicalism which was once the hallmark of the bolder forms of socialist thinking' (Giddens 1994: 73). Here we see the fundamental contradiction at the heart of Giddens' third way. On the one hand, he wants to break with the 'providentialism' (Giddens 1994: 249) of the left that argued that capitalism led to socialism, proletarians were the humanity's saviours and history had a clear direction. A complexity perspective would certainly agree with this position. On the other hand, his desire to find a radical 'new way' that gives the left back its position at the forefront of historical development has clear overtones of earlier 20th century attempts to create a linear order. Hence, by not recognising the full implications of complexity he opens up the third way to criticisms that it is both 'amorphous' and 'authoritarian' at the same time.

Giddens' reply to these critics is telling. For his 'amorphous' critics, he provides a bigger list of policies, desperately trying to reassert their newness and importance, while ignoring the charges of authoritarianism. A complexity perspective would agree with most of his flexible policy proposals, but argue that there is no clear policy answer to all situations. Beyond creating a stable fundamental order within which individuals can learn, interact and adapt, there is little a state can do. Moreover, complexity does not provide a moral framework for choosing between the different forms of social organisation. From a complexity perspective, one can argue that a society that is stable, open, democratic and encourages complex interaction is likely to be much more successful than a closed strictly ordered society, or a destabilised chaotic one. However, complexity cannot predict which type of similar societal organisation (the more market-oriented British, corporatistic Germans, socialistic Scandinavians etc) will be more successful than another. From a complexity framework, there are no certain strategies other than the most fundamental ones and as Dahrendorf (1999) stressed there are not three ways, but 100.

Regarding Giddens' continental critics who said they were already pursuing the third way, they are more correct than they know. From a complexity perspective, since there are so many possible 'ways', there is no particular reason why the US/UK, or any other state, should be seen as the leader of the third way. A particular set of strategies may work in one case, but not in another. One can make moral arguments over which system one may prefer, Scandinavian or British, but no state can claim to have the one and only 'way'. More fundamentally, there is no reason for the third way to be an inherently leftist strategy. A complexity framework implies uncertainty for both left and right. The two political movements have distinctive values that imply particular policy strategies. Nevertheless, they are both caught within the emerging complexity paradigm. Giddens' 'radical' desire to bring the left back to the 'forefront of history' betrays his inability to break with the earlier Newtonian framework. It may be politically appealing to the left, but is theoretically and practically unsustainable.

More specifically, in relation to the British welfare state, complexity theorists would be very sceptical of the audit and control culture that has emerged in response to the third way thinking of New Labour. In large and complex policy arenas, health, education and social policy, New Labour has striven to increase overall policy efficiency through a plethora of centrally driven targets that were designed to increase the effectiveness, responsiveness and oversight of policy provision. In essence, New Labour was treating these highly complex policy arenas as fundamentally linear mechanisms that could be controlled by centrally directed, hierarchical, command and control procedures. This position relied on the belief that political and administrative elites were in control of the policy arena, and that negative policy outcomes were merely a result of their lack of knowledge and control. Increase those and the policy should improve!

The clear problem, and a number of critics and commissions have made this point (Clarke *et al.* 2000), is that as the targets multiply they become increasingly detailed and increasingly difficult for the local actors to achieve. This is not due to local actor intransigence. In the NHS in 2003, hospital human resource managers are supposed to be responsible for over 330 targets! As one manager told us, because the targets influence each other (more resources to child-related diseases, influences waiting lists, staffing, maintenance, and so on) the most targets he could balance at one time were around 10! So, the obvious answer from an orderly linear perspective would be to hire more managers and give each of them 10 targets each. To a degree this is what New Labour has done in certain sectors of the health profession. The problem with this is that you cannot easily separate the targets into distinctive groups. The managers would still be stuck trying to coordinate 330 targets. And yet, despite these nearly impossible coordination tasks, the NHS continues to function on a daily basis providing a reasonable service for the 55 million British citizens. How can this be?

The answer is that the NHS (and education, economic and social policy arenas) is not a linear hierarchical structure, but an evolving complex adaptive one. As such, it easily fits within our complexity framework as demonstrated in Figure 4.3.

As we saw with the international system and EU, the NHS can easily be interpreted as a complex system composed of interacting orderly, disorderly and complex elements. Its core short-term framework, particularly its current basic resource parameters or allocations, rigidly determines the fundamental structure of the NHS. However, basic decisions over resource allocation already begin to introduce variation and unpredictability into the basic framework. Like grains of sand falling on a table shaping a generally stable, but constantly varying cone, the basic resource decisions to the various UK regions create a generally stable, but constantly varying output of health outcomes. Combine this with the continually evolving relationships between doctors, managers, consultants, nurses, etc and the debates over the very meaning of health and the health service, and you have a fundamentally complex adaptive system.

Likewise, a similar framework can be used for UK social policy in general as seen in Figure 4.4.

Again, it is the core short-term framework and basic resource parameters that set the most linear elements of UK social policy. This is then complicated by the complex dynamics of decisions over basic resources allocations, whether in relation to regional dynamics, struggles between different policy arenas (gender issues versus labour rights versus support for the disabled, etc) or other aspects. Institutional struggles between government departments, non-governmental organisations and local groups mirror the evolutionary dynamics of plant and

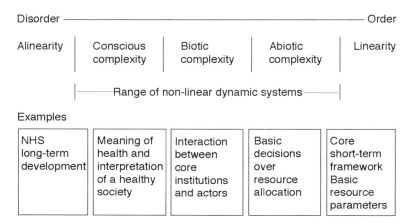

Figure 4.3 The range of NHS phenomena.

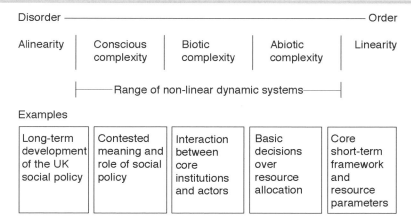

Figure 4.4 **The range of UK social policy.**

animal life in that their struggle over power resources and policy influence leads to the continual success and failure of certain groups, but a noticeable stability of the overall system. Meanwhile the narrative debates over the meaning and role of social policy are clear indications of conscious complexity. A brief glance at the history of social policy and evolution of its multiple meanings clearly demonstrates its contingent nature. Just think of the various and changing meanings of 'comprehensive school' in the post-WWII period. Finally, the long-term development of UK social policy, where it will be, what it will look like, how it will be debated, is clearly one of its most unpredictable and disorderly aspects. Clearly, as with Europeanisation, UK social policy can be conceived of as an evolving complex adaptive system. Once one makes this shift in thinking, the limits and dangers of more orderly 'third way' thinking become increasingly apparent.

Complexity and the EU–UK social policy relationship

Obviously, following on from the preceding sections it doesn't take much of an intellectual leap to insert the EU–UK social policy relationship into a complexity framework as demonstrated in Figure 4.5.

Again, the most stable and orderly elements of the EU–UK social policy relationship are the aspects of the core short-term framework. That interaction will occur, that neither side will end all interaction immediately and that embedded and institutionalised relationships will not vanish in the very short term are the most orderly, linear and predictable aspects of the relationship. These include aspects such as the relative weakness of EU–UK social policy relationship in relation to other policy areas, the controversial nature of that relationship to certain segments of the British public and the fundamental tension between more social inclusive continental social policy regimes and the more liberal UK regime. Shift to the basic power relationships between the core actors, whether it is the EU Commission interacting with the British Government, the British Parliament struggling to exert control over the departments or the Trades Union Congress (TUC) trying to use new EU labour legislation as a lever against the Confederation of British Industry (CBI), and one can see the probabilistic char-

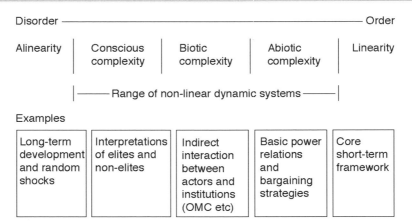

Figure 4.5 The range of EU–UK mechanisms of social policy interaction. OMC = open method of coordination.

acter of abiotic complexity. Move from the 'vertical' to the more 'horizontal' aspects of the relationship (such as the open method of coordination (OMC)) and one can easily see how emergence occurs in relation to policy development. Traditional social policy strategies were being blocked. Did the social actors merely stop what they were doing, collapse and go home? Of course not, they adjusted their strategies, evolved new tactics and a new emergent pathway was developed. In the category of conscious complexity, one merely needs to look at the evolution of the political parties' relationships to EU–UK social policies to glimpse the important role of narrative construction and debate. These party narratives have stable strands within them, but are continuously evolving and adapting in relation to political strategies, ideological beliefs and normative frameworks. For example, EU social policy has played a key role in helping to paste over the cracks in the Conservative Party's EU policy. It is the one area of EU policy that all Conservatives can agree to oppose. As such, it often becomes a convenient symbol for Conservative antagonism to the EU. Lastly, the most disorderly aspect of the relationship is the long-term framework and impact of random 'shocks'. As discussed earlier, it would have been virtually impossible to predict the state of EU–UK social policy interaction 20 or more years ago. If someone had stood up during a meeting of the Labour Party's National Executive Committee in the early 1980s and confidently predicted that Labour would soon become a unified pro-European party, they would have been certified insane! Similar predictions are equally difficult today. Predicting the nature of random events (the fall of communism in the USSR, the terrorist attacks of 11 September, even the tirade by the Italian Prime Minister Berlusconi against 'nazi' German Green Party Members of the European Parliament (MEPs)) and how they will impact on the relationship is one of the most disorderly aspects imaginable. And to tell the truth this is one of the main aspects that keeps the EU–UK social policy relationship interesting to watch.

So, if the EU–UK social policy relationship can be viewed from a complexity perspective what does this imply? First, in the context of our core question, the relationship between the EU and UK social policy relationship, linear, order-based and positivist methods can only tell part of the story as would a purely disorderly post-modernist approach. Second, general qualitative methods including historical pathways, institutional analyses, ideal-type modelling, semi-structured interviews, etc are central to capturing the complexity of most human phenomena. However, from a complexity perspective, the researcher must realise that he/she is viewing a part of a constantly evolving process and that their 'failure' to find the 'laws' of this relationship is a necessary outcome.

Does this mean that we can never make any real conclusions? No and Yes. For example, given all of this complexity, do the mechanisms of interaction that have been outlined in this chapter tend to encourage the centralisation or de-centralisation of UK social policy? The answer, not surprisingly, is: it depends. In general, the traditional mechanisms of policy interaction seem to increase the power of the Government and departments over the Parliament and social actors. They are the ones who are in direct contact with the EU, who make the deals at the EU level and who implement the policies. However, social actors have played a growing role in new policy areas and have played an active role in promoting new 'horizontal' forms of policy interaction. Where local actors have been of primary importance has been in the implementation of EU regional policy. Thus, the EU–UK social policy relationship exhibits both centralising and decentralising tendencies. Where this will lead in the future is very uncertain. Hence, the best we can do is use detailed studies within a broader framework to look for tendencies or patterns. This is exactly what the next four case study chapters will try to do!

Note

[1] An early example would come from China. Confucianism, which envisioned a strict social and moral code for society and the state, emerged out of an orderly period of Chinese dynastic history in the 6th century BC. Subsequent challengers, Buddhism and Taoism, thrived during periods of civil unrest and war during the 3rd to 6th centuries AD. Unsurprisingly, 'various attempts were made to harmonise the three schools of thought and to promulgate the idea that they were simply different ways by which to reach the same ultimate goal' (Smith 1973: 134). Consequently, one could argue that *san chiao* (the three religions or teachings) was the original third way.

Chapter 5

The European Employment Strategy and the UK: a case of coincidental convergence?

Of the various aspects of EU social policy, employment promotion is among its most important. However, this is only a recent phenomenon. In the 1950s and 1960s when West European unemployment rates hovered around 1–3%, employment matters were primarily the concern of the member states. During those years, the European Coal and Steel Community/European Economic Community (ECSC/EEC) focused on encouraging free movement of labour in order to lessen skill shortages and employment bottlenecks. With the growing unemployment of the 1970s and 1980s, European initiatives focused on employment protection rather than worker mobility. In the 1990s with the continued problems of long-term unemployment and the growing recognition of the diversity of the unemployment problem (Jackman 1998), the European Union (EU) shifted from employment protection to employment creation (Barnard 2000a; Biagi 2001). The centrepoint of this shift was the 1997 European Employment Strategy (EES), a rough compromise between the promotion of market-based job creation and social solidarity.

The EES was made possible not only by the emergence of a common consensus amongst the European Commission and several leading member states – including the UK – about the nature of Europe's employment challenges, but also by a significant change in regulatory approach. This shift in approach, reflecting a broader complexity shift in policy thinking, has seen a general transition from the promotion of hard laws (directives, regulations, etc) to the soft-regulatory procedures of the 'open method of coordination' (OMC) in employment strategies. The OMC emerged out of the 1997 Amsterdam Treaty revision and is 'based on policy guidelines, setting benchmarks, concrete targets and a monitoring system to evaluate progress via peer group reviews' (Barnard 2000a: 17). As such, the OMC has become an innovative new method of governance that has helped overcome practical and ideological barriers to European-level action through accommodating the heterogeneity that exists among the member states (Trubek and Mosher 2001a). Under the OMC complex common problems do not require simple common solutions.

In this chapter, we will explore how, despite a history of opposition to European employment initiatives, adapting to the EES has been easy for the British. This is largely because Britain already fared well in relation to many of the quantified objectives and, following the election of the Labour Government in May 1997, sought to develop and implement a programme of reform similar to that which was later advanced under the EES. Consequently, the UK was not required to significantly alter its existing policy approach in order to conform to the European requirements. Furthermore, where differences in policy approach have manifested themselves, the degree of adaptational pressure exerted by the non-binding procedures of the EES has, to date, proved relatively low. Hence, the EU–UK employment policy relationship is one of coincidental rather than planned convergence.

The chapter will conclude with a brief digression on the relationship between complexity theory and the development of the OMC.

The distinctiveness of UK and EU employment policies

As is well known, most people earn a living through selling their labour within the labour market (Moran 1994). National governments play an important role in regulating or deregulating these labour markets, determining the rights of employed persons and setting the overall level and structure of employment within the economy. In Britain, as elsewhere, the impact of the state on employment as a political issue increased significantly in the post-war period. During the immediate post-war years, the Attlee Labour Government developed a political programme based upon the economic teachings of Keynes and the social agenda of Beveridge that combined state responsibility for macroeconomic performance and full employment. The state's social duties were further developed through the creation of the welfare state, whereby it assumed greater responsibilities for education and training – thus strengthening the employability of individuals – and stronger welfare provision for those out of work. This commitment to maintaining full employment and an active welfare state set the framework of state employment and social policy for the next two decades.

However, this framework was increasingly undermined by the economic difficulties of the 1970s, seeing unemployment rise from around one million in 1975–1976, to two million in 1981 and over three million in 1984, and directly challenged by the election of Margaret Thatcher's right-wing Conservative Government in 1979. The change in government signified a fundamental ideological shift as the Conservatives pursued a neo-liberal agenda with an almost unwavering faith in the market's ability to deliver optimal economic and social conditions (Jones 1994). Such an approach inevitably precluded a commitment to the maintenance of full employment. While the Conservatives accepted the state still had a role in relation to issues of employment, they saw their primary responsibility as the creation of a sound macroeconomic environment through the adoption of monetarist policies to control inflation. In conjunction with these macroeconomic changes, the Conservatives saw a more limited role for social policy. While education and training continued to be regarded as essential for creating a qualified workforce, social regulations ultimately created more unemployment, not less (Jones 1994: 127). Economic recovery required the removal of these impediments to the market and reduction of state involvement in economic affairs (Kenner 1999: 39). At the time, high unemployment was seen as an acceptable price to pay for the return of a sound economy. In general, both the Major and Blair Governments have not radically departed from this emphasis on the expansion of market-led employment creation, rather than state-led employment rights.

As mentioned above, unemployment was not a significant problem for Europe in the 1950s and 1960s. When it grew in the 1970s and 1980s, most policy responses were nationally based. However, by the 1990s more and more effort was put into developing a European-level response. At that time, Europe was suffering from the effects of a low employment rate and high levels of unemployment. For example, in 1998 the employment rate for the 15 member states averaged 61.1%. Although this masked some considerable variations, for example Denmark and the UK enjoyed respective rates of 79.2% and 71.4% while Spain and Italy experienced rates of 50.2% and 51.8%, the EU average remained far lower than the 75% employment rate witnessed in the US (Larsson 1999: 7). Similarly, with 16.5 million people out of work in 1998 – one in ten of the EU workforce – Europe's unemployment rate was disappointing (European Commission 1999b: 3). Unemployment was not only high, but it exhibited a number of distinctive characteristics such as a high proportion of the jobless total experiencing long-term unemployment; half having been unemployed for more than one year with one-third for more than two years. Unsurprisingly, groups such as women, the young, the elderly, the disabled and ethnic minorities were all particularly disadvantaged (Meulders and Plasman 1997; European Commission 1999b: 3).

This was unacceptable to European-level actors for a number of reasons. Firstly, comparisons with the US demonstrated that if Europe could find the right mix of policies it could replicate the success of the US economy in translating growth into high levels of job creation. Data revealed that between 1993 and 1999, 81% of jobs created were paying above the median wage, thereby helping to dispel the myth that high US job creation levels were only in low paid jobs (HM Treasury 2002a: 85). Secondly, in the context of Europe's ageing population, the so-called 'demographic time-bomb', something had to be done to raise Europe's employment rate to improve public finances and make pension systems more sustainable (Barnard 2000a: 43). With the decline in the working age population already under way – beginning in Italy in 1999, Germany in 2001, and due to start in Britain in 2011 – an immediate response was required (Larsson 1999: 18). Thirdly, Europe's unemployment was exacting a high social cost for those individuals and communities affected, and contributing to unacceptable levels of poverty and social exclusion (European Commission 1999a: 3).

Despite the obvious diversity of member state economic dynamics and regimes, the European Commission identified two general causes at the heart of the European employment problem. The first was Europe's inability to handle macroeconomic shocks (European Commission 1999b) that accounted for a significant reduction in the EU's net growth in jobs. To rectify this situation the European Community has pursued a programme of macroeconomic reform through European Monetary Union (EMU) and efforts to complete the single market. However, macroeconomic shocks only explain part of the community's problems; a second cause was Europe's inability to handle transformations of the labour market (European Commission 1999b: 4). Structural deficiencies in Europe's labour market policies and social protection systems encouraged long-term unemployment, a factor identified as 'the core of Europe's employment failure' (Larsson 1999: 8). For the European Commission, with EMU gaining momentum in the economic sphere, something had to be done to modernise the 'European Social Model'.

However, while there was an emerging logic for the EU to play a growing role in combating European-wide employment problems, various factors militated against the Europeanisation of this policy area (Szyszczak 2000b; Trubek and Mosher 2001a). Traditionally, member states were reluctant to cede sovereignty/autonomy to the EU in this politically sensitive area. This reluctance was compounded by 'disparate national traditions' that were unsuitable for a 'traditional' harmonising approach based on 'hard' EU legislative directives and regulations (Ardy and Begg 2001). Further factors preventing the EU from developing a role in employment policy included: a weak treaty base prior to the Amsterdam revision, the emerging principle of subsidiarity and limited financial resources. In general, it was the conflict between the desire for a European-level employment policy and member state resistance that led to the creation and consolidation of the new and distinctive European Employment Strategy (EES).

EU developments from the EMU at Maastricht to the EES at Amsterdam

Between the signing of the Maastricht and Amsterdam Treaties the issue of employment rose to the top of the EU's political agenda helping unify the EU's economic and social policies into a single integrated approach. However, at Maastricht, the dichotomous nature of economic and social integration still persisted, and with economic policy clearly in the ascendancy, employment was only indirectly addressed.

At Maastricht the 12 heads of state and government agreed to a three-stage plan for EMU by 1999 at the latest. The plan followed a neo-liberal agenda in that it was believed a single currency would help maximise the benefits of a single market and create a stable macroeconomic platform for sustained growth and job creation. Therefore, while Maastricht did not develop a EU competence for employment policy per se, it did envisage that Europe's employment situation would improve due to the economic benefits provided by EMU. Debate had ensued as to whether employment should form part of the convergence criteria for EMU; however, the idea found little support among governments who were keen to guard their prerogatives in the field of employment policy. At this time the political space simply did not exist for the EU to develop a role in this area. However, as Europe's employment situation deteriorated further in the wake of Maastricht, it became increasingly evident that even if EMU could deliver macroeconomic stability, this would not prove the panacea to Europe's structural unemployment problems.

A further impetus for the Europeanisation of employment policy was provided by functional spillover from EMU (Ardy and Begg 2001: 4–7). Under a single currency the economies of the participating member states would become increasingly interdependent. This meant that the negative effects generated by a poor employment situation in any one country could have a detrimental impact on the eurozone as a whole (Sarfati 1998: 315). With a common monetary policy to be determined at the European level and constraints placed on national budgetary policies, employment policies 'could either be a by-product' of such decisions or form a 'core element' of the EU-level macroeconomic policy mix (Szyszczak

2000b: 199). Likewise, the 3% deficit limit imposed by the Stability and Growth Pact meant that countries may experience problems financing national welfare systems, especially when combined with ageing populations (Ardy and Begg 2001: 6). As such, EMU 'has led to the opening of new fields for discussion' at the European level (Pochet 1999: 277).

These developments provided the Commission with the political room to intensify its search for a new policy agenda to address Europe's mounting employment difficulties. In light of the changing economic and social environment, 'the Commission's challenge was to find a response that could preserve the essence of the European Social Model while creating the competitive conditions necessary to provide an estimated 15 million jobs' (Kenner 1999: 43). Between Maastricht and the treaty's revision at Amsterdam, the foundations for the current EES were laid through a series of high-level Commission publications. These successfully raised the issue of employment to the top of the Community's agenda and helped devise an appropriate form of governance that could overcome national resistance to European involvement in this sensitive area (Sciarra 1999: 158–160).

In the Commission's White Paper on *Growth Competitiveness and Employment*, an initial attempt was made to shift the emphasis away from employment rights to employment creation. It advocated:

> *thoroughgoing reform of the labour market, with the introduction of greater flexibility in the organisation of work and the distribution of working time, reduced labour costs, a higher level of skills, and pro-active labour policies* (European Commission 1993a: 124).

Yet although the White Paper raised the profile of employment at the European level significantly, it still approached the issue from a traditional neo-liberal perspective by viewing unemployment as the under-utilisation of an economic resource. This changed with the publication of the Green Paper, *European Social Policy: options for the Union*. Here, the Commission sought to develop a strategy designed to reconcile the economic need for job creation with the politics of social inclusion (European Commission 1993b; Barnard 2000a: 66). As the Green Paper proclaimed:

> *European social policy cannot be based on the idea that social progress must go into retreat in order for economic competitiveness to recover. On the contrary ... the Community is fully committed to ensuring that economic and social progress go hand in hand* (European Commission 1993b: 7).

Nevertheless, in searching for the 'right model' to run the European economy, the Commission still had to overcome problems associated with a limited treaty base for action, and national resistance to Europe assuming a traditional regulatory role in this area. The Commission resolved both these difficulties by advancing employment initiatives within the intergovernmental confines of the European Council (Kenner 1999: 48).

The member states responded to the Commission's 1993 White Paper at the Essen European Council in December 1994. The Council defined five priority areas that the member states were to address in their employment policies (*see*

Box 5.1). These recommendations were to be implemented through multi-annual programmes outlining national employment policies, and monitored jointly by the Commission and Council of Ministers. However, the 'Essen Process' had little direct impact, failing to convince the member states of the need to incorporate the 'Essen Priorities' into their adaptation programmes. As a result, 'few Member States attempted a coordinated European strategy to tackle unemployment' (Szyszczak 2000a: 202). However, Essen was significant in that it triggered a European-level discourse on the coordination of national employment policies. In so doing, Essen revealed a 'soft-law' trajectory along which employment policy could develop; one that could overcome the traditional barriers to the Europeanisation of this policy area.

Box 5.1   The Essen Priorities

The Essen Priorities recommended that member states:

- promote investment in vocational training
- increase employment intensive growth
- reduce non-wage labour costs
- improve the effectiveness of labour market policy
- tackle youth and long-term unemployment.

Title VIII of the Amsterdam Treaty represented a consolidation and extension of the 'soft law' developments within the field of employment policy during the preceding years. This compromise solution was to adapt the multilateral surveillance procedure, initially used in the EMU's Broad Economic Policy Guidelines, to coordinate labour market and welfare state reform. This procedure was based on a process of common guidelines, peer review and recommendations for corrective action.

> By adapting a similar approach for employment policy, it seemed possible to accommodate pressures for increased action at the EU level with contradictory pressure against expanding EU competence. The result was the Employment Chapter of the Amsterdam Treaty which formally created the EES (Trubek and Mosher 2001a).

From Luxembourg onwards: putting the guidelines into practice

At the special Luxembourg 'jobs summit' in November 1997 the Commission argued that the EU's unemployment problems stemmed from the inability of Europe's existing social model(s) to handle a combination of labour market transformation, technological change, economic globalisation and adverse demographic trends. Having been created in an earlier age to cater for the needs of a predominantly full-time male workforce, the national incarnations of the European Social Model were felt to be increasingly unable to cope with these modern developments. The Commission therefore argued that if European societies wished to raise employment levels while preserving their commitment to 'social solidarity' – a core factor underpinning the notion of a European Social Model (European Commission 1994) – then the member states needed to modernise their national welfare systems and labour market policies in response to these challenges (European Information Service (EIS) 2000: 23).

In practice, this translated into a need to tackle supply and demand side weaknesses within the labour market (Larsson 1999). On the supply side, weaknesses included low participation of older workers and women, high levels of long-term and regional unemployment, labour shortages in some regions and emerging skills gaps in certain sectors. Demand side weaknesses included high taxation on labour and the negative effect of red tape, particularly on small- and medium-sized enterprises (SMEs) (European Commission 2001b: 12). Together these factors contributed to relatively low levels of job creation during periods of growth, and significant job losses during periods of recession. Responding to these problems, the 'jobs summit' established a detailed four-pillar structure for the Employment Guidelines that became known as the 'Luxembourg Process' (*see* Box 5.2).

Box 5.2   The four pillars of the Luxembourg Process

1 **Employability Pillar.** To raise the employment rate the jobless need to have the right skills and incentives to work. Guidelines under this pillar seek to promote a *preventative approach* to combat long-term unemployment and an *activation approach* by moving policies towards supporting more active participation.

2 **Entrepreneurship Pillar.** Smaller companies represent one of the most dynamic areas of the economy. The pillar aims to exploit the employment and growth potential of SMEs by making it easier to start and run a business and employ people in it, reduce regulatory constraints and make the tax system more employment friendly.

3 **Adaptability Pillar.** In the context of globalisation and rapid technological change, modern business demands greater flexibility. The guidelines aim to encourage adaptability both for employees and businesses through the modernisation of work organisation and processes.

4 **Equal Opportunities Pillar.** The employment rate for women is far lower than the rate for men; furthermore, women face a range of other disadvantages in the labour market. The guidelines aim to address both issues through a gender mainstreaming approach across all the pillars, and promote policies aimed at tackling the gender gap, reconciling work and family life and facilitating re-integration into the labour market (Goetschy 2001: 402).

In response to the annual Employment Guidelines based around the four-pillar structure, and in accordance with the procedures contained under Article 128, the member states were required to submit annual national action plans (NAPs) that were then evaluated by the Council and Commission who then issued a joint evaluation report and, where necessary, formal Recommendations. The Luxembourg Process of planning, monitoring, examination and re-adjustment proved to be a popular format with around 20 Guidelines being issued each year.

While the process represents the main strand of the EU's coordinated approach to employment, subsequent summits have addressed other areas of employment-related policy. At the Cardiff and Cologne Summits in December 1998 and June 1999, Europe's national leaders agreed to launch two further 'processes' to promote employment. The 'Cardiff Process' outlined a soft regulatory strategy for 'comprehensive structural reforms and modernisation to improve the innovative capacity and efficiency of the goods, services and capital markets' (Council of the European Union 1998; Biagi 2001). Meanwhile, the 'Cologne Process' was initiated to improve the interaction between monetary, fiscal and wage policies (Council of the European Union 1999a). The Cologne Summit announced that these 'processes' and the earlier 'Luxembourg Process' constituted a 'European Employment Pact' (EEP). Overall, the creation of the EEP again demonstrated the shift in EU employment policy towards a coordination, rather than centralisation strategy.

Lisbon and beyond: broadening the EES agenda and process

While the EU has made significant progress in developing a coordinated employment strategy, a further extraordinary European Council was convened at Lisbon in March 2000 to strengthen the Community's agenda for economic and social reform. Consequently, although the agenda for the Lisbon Summit had a broader focus than employment, it nevertheless had significant implications for the development and broadening of the EES agenda.

The Lisbon Council was called on to develop a response to the challenges and opportunities of globalisation and the new 'knowledge-driven economy' (Council of the European Union 2000). To fulfil these aims the Lisbon Summit set the Union a new strategic goal for the next ten years:

> *to become the most competitive and dynamic knowledge-based economy in the world, capable of sustainable economic growth with more and better jobs and greater social cohesion.*

It was a rather broad and politically undivisive goal that emphasised the mutually reinforcing nature of economic, employment and social policies where economic reform must support employment and social cohesion, and social cohesion and high employment must sustain economic growth (Goetschy 2001: 405). In this respect, Europe's leaders at Lisbon endorsed a coherent 'triangulation' strategy that sought to overcome the political opposition and contradictions inherent within the Union's economic and social programmes of earlier years (European Commission 1999b: 13, 2000b).

The social dimension of the Lisbon agenda set out to modernise the European Social Model 'by investing in people' and 'developing a dynamic and active welfare state' (Council of the European Union 2000: 5). As such, Lisbon strengthened the EES by 'adopting the goal of full employment; setting medium-term employment targets and integrating the strategy into a wide framework of policy coordination' (European Commission 2002b: 2). The major quantified objectives for the Union are to raise the employment rate from an average of 61% (in March 2000) to 70% by 2010, and to increase the number of women in employment from an average of 51% to more than 60% over the same period. The result of this process has been that the employment rate target has become the 'central plank' in the Employment Strategy (Degryse and Pochet 2001: 13).

Regarding social security, due to fears over the long-term sustainability of public finances in the context of an ageing population, the Lisbon Summit also sought to modernise the EU's social protection systems. It called for greater cooperation between member states through the exchange of best practices, supported by a High Level Working Party on Social Protection mandated to examine the sustainability of pension systems up to 2020. Furthermore, Lisbon also acknowledged that the number of people living below the poverty line and in social exclusion was unacceptable, and emphasised that 'the best safeguard against social exclusion is a job' (Council of the European Union 2000). Hence, the EES became linked to both social security and exclusion.

To implement the Lisbon objectives, the European Council endorsed the use of the non-binding, soft-regulatory procedures of the 'open method of coordination' (OMC). At the time these methods were already in use in several policy fields such as employment (through the 'Luxembourg Process'), structural economic reform (the 'Cardiff Process'), and macroeconomic policy (the Broad Economic Policy Guidelines (BEPGs)) (Goetschy 2001: 406). Although the precise nature of these processes varied, they all used a range of coordinating techniques including the setting of European Guidelines, the use of quantitative and qualitative indicators and benchmarks, the submission of national and/or regional implementation reports, and periodic monitoring, evaluation and peer review (Degryse and Pochet 2001: 13). However, the Lisbon Summit sought to extend the use of these procedures to a further range of policy areas associated with the transition to a knowledge economy, education policy and lifelong learning, and the fight against social exclusion (Goetschy 2001: 406). To further define the relevant mandates under these procedures and ensure they are being followed up, Lisbon also established a stronger role for the European Council in 'guiding', 'coordinating' and 'monitoring' the process of reform (Council of the European Union 2000). As such, an additional meeting of the European Council devoted to economic and social affairs is now held every spring with the intention of ensuring greater coherence between the policies pursued within this field.

Most recently, the European Employment Guidelines have been modified to reflect the priorities expressed in the Council's conclusions. The main innovation was the introduction of 'horizontal objectives' that overarch the detailed four-pillar structure of the Luxembourg Process. These require member states to *consider* setting national targets for raising the rate of employment in order to reach the overall employment targets established at Lisbon. Following the annual Spring Council on economic and social affairs in Stockholm in March 2001, new intermediate targets were included in the 2002 Guidelines to increase the overall employment rate to 67% by 2005 and employment rate for women to 57%. In addition a new employment rate target of 50% for older persons (aged between 55 and 64 years) was established for 2010. Further horizontal objectives call on the member states to maintain and improve 'quality in work', develop comprehensive and coherent strategies for lifelong learning, develop a comprehensive partnership with the social partners for the implementation, monitoring and follow-up of the Employment Strategy, set their priorities in a balanced manner in order to respect the integrated nature and equal value of the Guidelines, and strengthen the development of common indicators in order to evaluate progress under all four pillars (Council of the European Union 2001c; Council of the European Union 2002b).

Is the EES compatible with the 'third way'?

As discussed above, between the Maastricht and Amsterdam Treaty revisions the Union's conception of its role in economic and social policy underwent a fundamental paradigm shift. Through the creation of the EES, the EU was able to overcome many of the earlier antagonisms between its economic and social dimensions and forge a new policy framework. Furthermore, by focusing on employment the EU was able to unite a range of previously ring-fenced and *ad hoc* Union competencies (especially in relation to social policy) and extend its influence into a number of policy areas traditionally seen as the sole prerogative of the nation-state. In so doing, the Union was able to transcend much of the ideological polarity that had previously existed within this field and create a more coherent economic and social agenda which, a number of commentators have argued, is synonymous with the 'third way' (Kenner 1999; Biagi 2001).

However, despite Giddens' claims as to the newness of his 'third way', the notion of a 'third' or 'middle way' between polarised left–right strategies has been a recurring feature in the programmes of predominantly left-wing parties during earlier times and in a number of countries. Most recently, during the 1990s, policies based on a reconciliation between left- and right-wing strategies found favour in other major European capitals with the election of centre-left parties in both Germany – under Gerhard Schröder – and Italy – under the future Commission President Romano Prodi. The Commission had also been employing the language of the 'third way', in various publications between the Maastricht and Amsterdam Treaty revisions, in its search for a new model to respond to the many challenges confronting Europe (Kenner 1999: 39–47). Over time, these ideas coalesced into the agenda of the European Employment Strategy. Therefore, as Kenner observed, while 'the Third Way has provided a convenient label for a forward looking agenda' and is 'most often associated with Blair and other revisionist leaders such as Schröder and Prodi', it has also been 'resonant in the thinking of the Community's actors over the past decade' (Kenner 1999: 47). The emergence of a 'third way' coincidental consensus among the Commission and a number of leading member states thus enabled the EU to develop a coordinated employment strategy. In this consensus, instead of playing its typical role of isolated and reluctant EU employment policy actor, Britain found itself at the heart of this new European economic and social agenda.

Moreover, the EES' use of innovative 'management by objectives approach based on the use of guidelines, benchmarks and systematic monitoring' (Brunn 2001: 314) is in many ways much more open than the more linear aspects of Giddens' third way. In particular, the open method of coordination promotes interaction among states whereby each country is able to find the appropriate mix of policies suitable for their stage of development and political orientation, subject to a series of commonly agreed objectives. As Tucker identified, 'The essence of the process is to identify common ends without common means' (Tucker 2000: 71). Thus, instead of trying to find the new uniform way for European employment policy, the EES provides a flexible target-based strategy that offers the member states, and a range of other policy actors, considerable scope for obtaining common objectives through distinctive strategies.

This is not to say that the EES is a completely open-ended disorderly process. For example, there are quantified targets[1] in the European Guidelines, albeit ones stemming from 'soft law' rather than binding measures contained within the treaty. In these areas Biagi (1998: 326) argues 'one cannot speak simply of coordination; a policy of convergence would be more correct'. Moreover, as the Luxembourg Process has evolved over successive European Summits, the number of Guidelines that contain quantified targets has increased, placing further obligations on member states to converge towards centrally agreed aims (Biagi 2001). However, irrespective of this trend, the majority of Guidelines remain broad and do not specify quantified objectives. Furthermore, 'to the extent that the EES does seek convergence it is often a convergence of outcomes, not of policies'. Where targets *are* established the member states are allowed to 'choose the best means to reach those results' (Trubek and Mosher 2001a: 6.4). Finally, where the Guidelines have been quantified, since the Council must approve these Guidelines, these are the areas for which there is generally broad political support for such targeting.

For the UK in general, these fundamental targets were easily met without the Government having to significantly alter its existing policy approach. As de la Porte (2002: 56) has argued, although as a method of governance the EES/OMC is intended to 'respect national practices, discourses, and frames of reference', it does imply more fundamental structural alterations for some countries. In this respect, the EES has proved most suited to those countries that were already performing well in relation to the employment targets, or who were undertaking the type of reforms advocated under the strategy. Given the similar coincidental convergence between new Labour's 'third way' and the Commission's new agenda for economic and social policy reform, complying with the EES has required lower levels of policy adaptation in Britain than most other member states which occasionally required a '180-degree turn to adapt to all four pillars' of the EES (de la Porte 2002: 48). But despite this general ease of adaptation, were particular elements of the EES difficult to integrate into UK employment policy?

Applying the EES pillars in the UK: variations within an evolving framework

Assessing the impact of the EES on the UK is problematic due to the primarily indirect (horizontal) impacts of the EES on UK employment policy. Hence, it

> cannot be measured in traditional terms, that is, under a sort of coercive perspective ... [it] must be assessed in the long run, with special reference to single aspects of labour market and industrial relations regulations (Biagi 2001: 161).

This difficulty is intensified by the division of the EES into four separate policy pillars: employability, entrepreneurship and job creation, encouraging adaptability and equal opportunities (*see* Box 5.2). In order to assess the impact of these pillars, this section will briefly review the main objectives of the first three pillars (exploring the fourth pillar in Chapter 6) and then use the UK's annual Employment Action Plans and Joint Employment Reports to review the British policy response to these developments. In addition it will also address concerns that the EES simply leads to a 'repackaging of existing policies' rather than genuine policy change (Ardy and Begg 2001: 12–13). Finally, and perhaps most importantly in assessing the degree of adaptational pressure exerted by this process, it will assess how the UK has responded to the non-binding Council Recommendations issued under Article 128.4 of the Treaty. These instances provide an opportunity to assess how the Government responds when weaknesses in Britain's initial policy approach have been identified.

A comparison of the pillars will show that the impact of the EES on the UK has been uneven across the pillars (European Commission 2001d: 6; Trubek and Mosher 2001a: 11). Attention has focused on measures to develop employability, followed by efforts to promote 'entrepreneurship'. This can be explained by the fact that both areas were already central to the Labour Government's agenda for modernising labour market and welfare policies on their accession to office in 1997. By contrast the Government's measures to promote the adaptability of businesses and their employees reveal a number of differences between the British and European approaches.

Pillar I: improving employability – reinforcing coincidental convergence

The main policy objectives of the Employability Pillar are to raise the employment rate and tackle youth and long-term unemployment. Over the five-year cycle of the EES, the Guidelines have sought to realise these aims, predominantly through a combination of:

- comprehensive tax-benefit reforms
- active, rather than passive, labour market policies for the unemployed and inactive
- lifelong learning strategies designed to provide skills for the new labour market
- efforts to promote social inclusion.

Measures to improve 'employability' have formed the cornerstone of the Labour Government's employment policy since 1997. Mirroring many of the priorities addressed under the Employability Guidelines, the Government has formulated and implemented a series of reforms that seek to 'make work pay' and 'make work possible' (Department for Education and Employment (DfEE) *et al.* 2001: 1.5–8). Policies to improve education and training have also featured prominently on the Government's agenda, while social inclusion has been highlighted as 'an intrinsic element of all its policies' (ECOTEC Research and Consulting 2002: 41).

Tax and benefit reforms are also central to the Government's commitment to 'make work pay' by tackling financial disincentives to work. Unemployed people are understandably reluctant to take up work if it makes them worse off. To rectify this situation the Government introduced a package of reforms, initially announced in the 1998 Budget, designed to increase the returns that can be obtained by working compared to remaining on welfare. These measures included new tax credits to deliver extra help to those on low and moderate incomes,[2] reforms to the system of National Insurance Contributions (NICs), changes to the rate at which income tax is levied[3] and the introduction of a national minimum wage[4] (DfEE *et al.* 2001; HM Treasury 2001: 17).

Linked to these new incentives, the Labour Government has devised a number of active labour market policies designed to 'make work possible'. The core measure for reconnecting the unemployed with the workforce is the Jobseekers' Allowance (JSA) that combines benefit payments with active jobsearch measures. Already in operation before the 1998 Guidelines, all recipients of the JSA receive intensive jobsearch assistance in the form of an individualised job plan from their first day of unemployment (Tucker 2000: 73). Thereafter, claimants must further demonstrate they are both available for and actively seeking work at fortnightly meetings. While the majority of people are known to find work relatively quickly, some require greater assistance. This is predominantly provided through the Government's New Deal initiatives.

The New Deal for Young People (NDYP), launched in April 1998, is targeted at all 18–24 year olds who have been claiming JSA for six months or longer. It aims to tackle youth unemployment and prevent the flow of this group into long-term unemployment. The programme begins with the New Deal Gateway whereby each participant receives intensive help, tailored to the needs of the individual, initially through a period of counselling, advice and guidance lasting up to four months. Those who do not find work during this period may be offered subsidised employment for six months, or up to 12 months' training without loss of benefit (DfEE 1998: 9–11). This programme has been followed by a similar *mandatory* New Deal for people aged 25 plus (ND25plus), initially designed to help adults who had been unemployed for two years or more. Again, this offers six months of subsidised employment or training for up to one year, for those who are unable to find work after an initial period of intensive jobsearch assistance (DfEE 1998: 10–11). Further *voluntary* New Deal programmes have since been introduced to help other vulnerable groups in society. These include: a New Deal for the Over-50s (ND50plus) that builds on the existing provisions of the ND25plus (DfEE 1999: 14); a New Deal for Lone Parents and a New Deal for Partners of Unemployed People, both designed primarily to help women return to the labour market; and a New Deal for Disabled People. This aims to assist those with a disability or long-term sickness

move from Incapacity Benefit or Severe Disablement Allowance into employment (DfEE 2000: 12).

A further prominent strand in the UK's 'welfare to work' programme is the
commitment to developing a 'learning society' in which everyone will be
expected to learn and upgrade their skills throughout life (Tucker 2000: 74).
This Lifelong Learning Strategy is seen to be particularly important response to
the increasing challenges of the labour market and to improving the UK's weak
skills base in relation to her main international competitors (HM Treasury *et al.*
2002: 69). In Britain, 7 million adults lack basic literacy and numeracy skills,
amounting to 24% of the adult population (ECOTEC Research and Consulting
2002: 38). Evidence of recruitment difficulties experienced by UK employers
due to a shortage of specialist IT skills is also causing concern. In response to
these weaknesses the Government has overseen a significant increase in public
expenditure on education and training,[5] and introduced a number of initiatives
designed to promote adult learning including Learndirect, the Learning and
Skills Council and Individual Learning Accounts (DfEE *et al.* 2001; Department
for Work and Pensions (DWP) 2002).

Finally, employment measures to promote social inclusion also feature
prominently on the Government's agenda. The socially excluded refers to
groups and individuals who experience particular disadvantage in the labour
market such as the disabled, ethnic minorities and the elderly. The 2001 Green
Paper: *Towards Full Employment in a Modern Society* established the Government's
target to improve social inclusion by closing the gap in employment rates for
these excluded groups and areas by 2004 (DfEE *et al.* 2001: 2). In attaining this
target, the mainstream employment and training measures discussed above,
such as tax-benefit reforms, active labour market policies and lifelong learning
strategies, form a key part of the Government's approach. This is 'based on the
principle that jobs offer the best route out of social exclusion' (DWP 2001: 18).
In a number of instances these measures were specifically tailored to serve the
needs of socially excluded groups. For example, the NDYP, ND25plus and the
New Deal for Lone Parents were structured to actively promote equality of
opportunity and outcome for individuals from ethnic minorities. In particular,
since its launch in January 1998, the NDYP monitored in detail the ethnicity of
its participants 'to ensure that ethnic minorities are as successful in finding
work as their white peers' (DWP 2001: 19). Similarly, the Government targeted
the disabled and elderly through the New Deal for Disabled People and
ND50plus programmes. These measures were accompanied by a range of more
specific initiatives including the creation of the Disability Rights Commission in
1999 and the introduction of a Code of Practice on Age Diversity in
Employment.

Not surprisingly, given all of these new employment initiatives since 1997,
the UK met all of the objectives of the Employability Pillar Guidelines
(European Commission 2002b: 25). Since 1998, all the annual Joint
Employment Reports noted that Britain placed the greatest emphasis on developing 'employability' measures within its annual Employment Action Plans
(EAPs). The European Council and Commission acknowledged that these
measures are removing financial disincentives to work. The UK is felt to be
performing well in respect of the EU-wide target of cutting the inflow of young
people and adults into long-term unemployment (European Commission

2001d). In the first Joint Employment Report (JER) published in 1998 the UK's NDYP was identified as an example of 'good practice', for moving policies for the unemployed from a passive to an active basis, and highlighted that the Government established ambitious targets for promoting lifelong learning to address low levels of basic skills (European Commission 2000e).

However, despite this high degree of convergence, there is little evidence to suggest that the Guidelines were a significant factor in shaping Britain's 'employability' policies. A large number of these initiatives were included within the Labour Party's 1997 election manifesto, adopted from policy reforms in the USA (Dolowitz and Marsh 1996) and implemented before the first round of Employment Guidelines was issued in 1998. In many instances the Government was thus able to demonstrate compliance with the European Guidelines simply by including details of existing initiatives within the UK's annual EAP. This is most evident in relation to the NDYP. The NDYP was a core element of the 1997 manifesto and was launched before the first Guidelines were issued. Following the scheme's articulation within the 1998 EAP, the New Deal was identified as an example of 'good practice' in the subsequent JER (European Commission 1999b: 38). Likewise, whilst the comprehensive tax-benefit reforms in the Government's 'Making Work Pay' package were commended in the 2001 JER for improving the 'incentive structures, reinforcing control systems and tightening eligibility conditions' (European Commission 2001d: 22), these too were announced prior to the publication of the first round of Guidelines. As such, the annual Employment Guidelines did not induce significant domestic policy adaptation in this field. At most, one could argue that the Guidelines had a reinforcing effect on UK employment policies.

On the other hand, despite the close approximation between the British and European policy objectives for improving 'employability', Britain *has* received recommendations for urgent action under the Employability Pillar in accordance with Treaty Article 128. In 2001, following the joint surveillance of Britain's EAP, the Government received two formal Council Recommendations. These Recommendations were essentially repeated in 2002. The first Recommendation stated that the UK should:

> *Reinforce active labour market policies for the adult unemployed before the 12 month point, so as to increase the number of people benefiting from active measures, and supplement the support provided by the Jobseekers' Allowance Regime* (Council of the European Union 2001b).

In both years the Council, acting on a Recommendation from the Commission, concluded that Britain had failed to comply with the obligation to offer unemployed adults a 'new start' before reaching 12 months of unemployment. Under the common European indicator for this Guideline, the 2001 JER argued that only 14.2% of the unemployed participated in an 'active measure', thereby falling well short of the 20% target required (European Commission 2002d: 102). While the JER acknowledged that further support was available at 12 months it felt that 'the interaction of the JSA active benefit and more active support for more people at 12 months would provide a fully coherent preventative approach' (European Commission 2001c: 213). Moreover, with unemployment so low, those reaching the New Deal at 18 months are the most hard to help and less able to compete in the labour market (European Commission 2001d: 85). Therefore, the EU observed that most unemployed adults did not receive intensive support until after 24 months when they moved on to the ND25plus, which was deemed inconsistent with Guideline 1 (2001 and 2002) on preventing long-term unemployment.

Although the British Government partially responded to this Recommendation by bringing forward the point of intervention to 18 months, from the initial point of two years, this still falls short of the 12-month date envisaged under the Guidelines. However, in both the 2001 and 2002 EAPs, the Government forcibly argued that the JSA is an active, rather than passive, unemployment benefit system. As such it provides *all* unemployed people with active jobsearch assistance from their first day of unemployment in accordance with the Guidelines, with additional assistance becoming available after 6 and 12 months of unemployment prior to the New Deal. Furthermore, the Government claimed that the structure of the UK labour market, with its rapid movement into and out of employment, renders the introduction of large-scale assistance for the adult unemployed before 12 months inappropriate. As such it argued further intervention would prove costly and 'distance jobseekers from the labour market', thereby reducing their chances of finding work quickly (DfEE 2001: 8–9). In consequence, the Government has failed to significantly adapt UK policy in response to the Council Recommendation, all the while insisting that the UK's existing policy framework fully conforms to the Guideline and has 'one of the lowest proportions of long-term unemployed in the EU' (DWP 2002: 9).

Overall, EU–UK policy interaction under Pillar I is one of reinforcing coincidental convergence. New Labour's employability strategies were well developed before the creation of the Guidelines and very similar to the general approach of the Guidelines. Minor divisions remain, but overall their coincidental convergence probably reinforces Labour Party employability strategies within the UK.

Pillar II: developing entrepreneurship and job creation – vague convergence

Similar to Pillar I, Pillar II has not been problematic for UK policy. The entrepreneurship pillar aims to generate conditions favourable for the creation of new jobs (European Commission 2001d: 27). For the Labour Government, the development of an enterprise culture is a key objective of UK employment policy and central to improving the domestic employment situation. From the outset, British policies towards promoting entrepreneurial activity were similar to those advanced at the European level. The Labour Government's emphasis on small businesses and the creation of the Small Business Service (April 2000) to 'act as a voice for small business and improve the coherence and quality of Government support for small businesses' (Tucker 2000: 76), is a clear parallel to the EU's emphasis on small and medium sized enterprises (SMEs). The Government has also taken steps to reduce both bureaucratic red tape and overall tax burdens on SMEs, reducing tax for small companies by nearly 25% making Britain's the lowest starting rate among major industrialised countries (DfEE 2001: 21) and giving the UK 'one of the shortest lead-in times for starting a new business and the second lowest rate of non-wage labour costs in the EU' (European Commission 2000c; 2001: 211).

Already recognised as one of the best performers in terms of employment in services, the Government is committed to building on this reputation by making the UK 'the best location in the world for e-commerce by 2002'. This is to be achieved by removing barriers to e-commerce and introducing tax breaks to encourage investment in information computer technology (ICT) (European Commission 2000c). The UK's strategy to promote entrepreneurship and job creation is also increasingly being pursued at the regional and local level through the English Regional Development Agencies (RDAs) and Regional Action Plans that cover 'delivery of objectives through partnership, the encouragement of employment initiatives, development of local labour markets, and stimulation of entrepreneurship' (DfEE 2001: 22).

These objectives are broadly in line with the Community Guidelines under the Entrepreneurship Pillar, and successive JERs have recognised Britain's compliance with these Community objectives. However, the Guidelines under the Entrepreneurship Pillar are far broader and less demanding than those regarding employability and do not contain quantified targets. For example, in 2001 Guideline 12 stated:

> *Each Member State will set a target*, if necessary *and taking account of its present level, for gradually reducing the overall tax burden, and* where appropriate, *set a target for gradually reducing the fiscal pressure on labour and non-wage labour costs* ... (Council of the European Union 2001c) [emphasis added].

In response to this Guideline the UK chose not to set such a target (DfEE 2001: 24). To date no Council Recommendations have been issued to Britain under Pillar II. Therefore, while Britain adequately fulfils the objectives contained under the Entrepreneurship Pillar, the UK has, again, not had to significantly modify her existing policy approach in order to comply with the European Guidelines. Consequently, EU–UK convergence on Pillar II is due primarily to the vagueness of the pillar and the general compatibility between EU–UK policy regimes. Overall, Pillar II has had a very limited impact on entrepreneurial policy.

Pillar III: encouraging adaptability of businesses and their employees – adjustment without convergence

The aim of the Adaptability Pillar is to modernise the organisation of work to respond to the competitive demands of a globalised and knowledge-based economy. The Guidelines focus on reconciling the need for greater flexibility in working arrangements, with the need to ensure job security. Given that much of this 'adaptation' is required at the level of the workplace, the Pillar's Guidelines demand that the social partners, in conjunction with national Governments, play a leading role in fostering this process of modernisation. In recent years the Pillar has also given a greater emphasis to promoting the adaptability of employees within enterprises, notably by calling upon the social partners to develop strategies for lifelong learning. Few of the Guidelines contained under the Adaptability Pillar contain quantified objectives.

Since Labour's accession to office in 1997, many of the main priorities addressed under the Adaptability Pillar have, again, broadly coincided with the Government's employment relations' agenda (ECOTEC Research and Consulting 2002: 62). However, Labour has been very reluctant to adopt more continental-style labour regulations. Since the first EAP was submitted in 1998, it has stressed the high degree of UK labour market flexibility, and continually argued that the individualistic nature of employment contracts within the UK labour market enables both employers and workers:

> to adopt the type of work organisation and practice which best suits their individual needs and circumstances [and leads to a] 'highly diverse and adaptable range of working practices' in the UK (DfEE 2000: 22).

For example only a third of UK employees work a 'standard' week of between 35 and 40 hours compared to over 60% in the EU as a whole (DfEE 1998: 30).

At the same time the Government has recognised that such a flexible system needs to be balanced with a complementary 'framework of minimum standards of fairness' within the workplace (DfEE 2000: 23). For example, the Employment Act 2002 gave parents with young children the right to request flexible working arrangements following a recommendation from the Work and Parents Taskforce. More importantly, following the decision of the newly elected 1997 Labour Government to sign the Social Chapter, a host of changes have been introduced in response to recent European Directives such as protection for workers on part-time and fixed-term contracts from unequal treatment, new statutory limits on working time, and new entitlements to parental and maternity leave.

In addition to these legislative changes, the Government has sought to improve levels of adaptability within the workplace and labour market through its broad commitment to lifelong learning and workplace partnership (DfEE 2001; DfEE *et al.* 2001). As such, the Government has sought to foster new forms of partnership in workplace and policy-making process in order to move away from 'old confrontational structures' (Tucker 2000: 78; ECOTEC Research and Consulting 2002: 62). However, these reforms were made within the general framework of the UK's long-established tradition of negotiating agreements at company or workplace level, rather than using the regional or national level bargaining that occurs in most other member states (DfEE 2001: 7). Hence, these changes have not significantly altered the UK's more voluntarist industrial relations system where discussions between employers and trade unions on issues such as wages and contracts are typically handled at the local level 'without direct government involvement' (DfEE 2000: 2, 8).

In reviewing the UK's annual EAPs, the Council and Commission have formally recognised the progress made by the UK since 1997 in 'establishing a framework of minimum standards in the workplace' (European Commission 2002e: 277). However, these reforms owe little to the European Guidelines of the Adaptability Pillar. Instead they are the combined result of a nationally inspired agenda for labour market reform and the European Directives adopted since the Maastricht Treaty revision. So while a number of these policy changes are attributable to the forces of vertical Europeanisation, this stems from the EU's 'hard' law Directives rather than the soft-regulatory procedures of the Adaptability Guidelines.

The UK's oppositional attitude towards social partnership compared to most other member states highlights the differences between the UK's approach to labour relations and that of the Adaptability Guidelines. Thus, Britain has received Recommendations urging greater social partnership in 2000, 2001 and 2002 that did lead to a number of incremental changes in Britain's approach towards partnership strategies. In 2000 and 2001 Council Recommendations urged Britain:

to enable the social partners at all levels to reach agreements on the moderni-sation of work organisation (Council of the European Union 2000)

and foster 'social partnership at all appropriate levels' (Council of the European Union 2001b).

In response to these criticisms, the Government, Confederation of British Industry (CBI) and Trades Union Congress (TUC) established a range of initia-tives. Most notably the Partnership Fund was set up to 'support organisations who are committed to working in partnership with employees to solve business issues and to develop better employment relations within the workplace' (DWP 2002: 38). Government funds were also made available under the Union Learning Fund to encourage trade unions to support learning opportunities for their members (Tucker 2000: 78). The JERs have since acknowledged the 'strong role of partnership at the local level' (European Commission 2001d: 84), by stating 'local partners have been given an increasingly powerful and flexible role in tackling problems, especially policies for lifelong learning' (European Commission 2001d: 212).

More broadly, the Labour Government now claims to work closely with the Social Partners in formulating national regulations to implement European Directives, 'particularly those based on Social Partner agreements' (DfEE 2001: 27; DWP 2002: 39–40), and in the development of the UK's annual EAP, making a direct contribution to the 1998, 1999 and 2000 Plans. In October 2001 at the behest of the Government, the CBI and TUC published their joint report on 'The UK Productivity Challenge'. Since then, the CBI and TUC have agreed to continue to work together to take forward this agenda, with a particular focus on raising the level of basic skills. The TUC and CBI are also active on the Learning and Skills Council, the Work and Parents' Taskforce and the Teleworking Working Group. Finally, in addition to these 'flexible task-focused groups', the TUC and CBI are represented on a number of permanent bodies including the Advisory Conciliation and Arbitration Service (ACAS), the Health and Safety Commission and the Low Pay Commission (LPC).

Despite these changes, EU actors remain critical of the UK approach to labour relations. For example, although the European Council and Commission recog-nised the 'strengthened role for the UK's two major National Social Partners' over the period (DfEE 2001: 84), they acknowledge that the UK approach 'remains to consult Social Partners on policy implementation "where appropri-ate" with no general framework for their involvement' (DWP 2002: 101). Furthermore, the Social Partners continue to remain 'less involved in actual delivery' (European Commission 2001d: 211). Most recently the 2002 Council issued a Recommendation urging the UK to:

further foster social partnership at the national *level to improve policy imple-mentation and development. In particular, efforts should be aimed at improving productivity and skills, and the modernisation of working life* (Council of the European Union 2002c) [emphasis added].

Overall, the Guidelines and Recommendations issued under the Adaptability Pillar have induced a degree of domestic policy adaptation in relation to the way the Social Partners are involved in the modernisation of work organisation and improving productivity and skills. However, the current Labour Government had already expressed a similar commitment to fostering new forms of partner-ship in order to promote adaptability within the labour market. The EES can therefore be seen as helping to facilitate this process of domestic reform, rather than foisting a fundamental policy transformation upon a reluctant British Government. As such the Social Partners have become more closely involved in policy delivery at the enterprise, local, regional *and* national level. However, at the national level the Labour Government has resisted demands to alter the basically conflictual nature of the UK's traditional decentralised and voluntarist industrial relations system (European Commission 2002a: 278). Adjustments have been made, but no convergence.

Conclusion

In recent years, evidence of unacceptably high and persistent levels of un-employment, caused by significant structural weaknesses in Europe's existing economic and social models has prompted the Commission and member states to search for ways of addressing these common challenges. This general problem has helped forge a more cohesive economic and social agenda than previously existed at the European level and opened up a number of new policy areas to EU initiatives. However, given that attempts to tackle Europe's employ-ment difficulties require reform in some of the most politically sensitive and institutionally divergent areas of national policies (Szyszczak 2000a, 2000b), a new method of governance was required. Accordingly the European Employment Strategy became the foundation for the innovative 'open method of coordination' approach.

The principal advantage of this form of governance is that it provides 'the means towards common solutions to common problems without demanding the sort of harmonisation that would be anathema to many governments' (Ardy and Begg 2001: 11). The flexibility inherent within the system allows govern-ments to tailor reforms to their own situations while remaining within the context of a coordinated European framework. As Janine Goetschy (2000) observed, the EES encourages a simultaneous 'Europeanisation' and a 're-nationalisation' of employment policies. Having integrated the European Council and Commission into the policy-making process, the primary responsi-bilities of the EU under the EES are to 'construct the broad strategy, develop specific guidelines, monitor performance, and call for periodic adjustments' (Trubek and Mosher 2001b: 6.1). By contrast, the member states continue to determine the detailed content of domestic employment policy (European Commission 2001b: 7). In this respect, the EES merely serves as 'one of a number of forces impinging on domestic policy-makers' (Trubek and Mosher 2001a: 13).

While the EES is comprised of a number of dimensions and processes, the main element of this coordinated strategy is the Luxembourg Process and although evaluating the impact of the Process on domestic employment policies is complicated by the specific nature of its soft-regulatory procedures, one can draw some general conclusions. First, the UK has not had to modify its fundamental employment or industrial relations policy approach significantly in order to comply with many of the aims of the EES. This is most noticeable in relation to the overall and female employment rate targets contained under the horizontal objectives, but is also true of many of the specific Employment Guidelines – particularly those under the Employability and Entrepreneurship Pillars. Thus, although the EES has required the member states to converge towards a number of common employment targets, the fact that the UK has continuously exceeded these targets has meant the UK has not had to contemplate major reforms in order to attain them. Similarly, the 'third way' programme of labour market and welfare reform advanced by Labour since 1997 largely coincided with the main principles of reform put forward by the EES (European Commission 2002b). These similarities have served to limit the degree of domestic policy adaptation required for the UK to comply with many of the European Guidelines. As a result, Britain has fared well during the process of peer review simply by repackaging existing policies.

Second, where differences have existed between the requirements of the EES and existing British policy, the Guidelines and non-binding Council Recommendations have exerted a relatively low level of adaptational pressure. Having received a number of formal Recommendations, minor adaptations can be detected in relation to the UK's policies towards social partnership and childcare. However, these are areas in which the Labour Government had already expressed a prior commitment to reform. As such, the EES merely reinforced earlier UK policy strategies. In contrast, where the EES challenged the fundamentally voluntary nature of the UK industrial relations system, British Government chose to ignore repeated Council Recommendations by claiming its existing policy framework already complied with EES requirements. This demonstrates that the UK has only taken on board the Council Recommendations where these have been broadly in line with the national programmes of reform (de la Porte 2002: 56). Thus, forces of Europeanisation exerted by the EES have, to date, only contributed to a process of uneven incremental change in British employment policy.

In this respect, the influence of the EES should been seen more in terms of fostering political agreement on 'new common paradigms', such as lifelong learning and quality in work (European Commission 2002b), rather than fundamentally overhauling the minutiae of domestic employment and industrial relations policies. This process of uneven incremental change in UK employment policy is the sort of change that the new OMC should be expected to produce: a new form of complex governance evolving in response to the sensitivity and complexity of the employment policy process it was designed to manage.

Final point: complexity and the open method of coordination

Although one can find elements of complex adaptational and emergent activity throughout the EU–UK employment policy relationship, how can complexity help one to understand a specific element of that relationship? A good example of the usefulness of complexity can be found in the development of the OMC. For commentators from traditional perspectives where one must have clear lines of authority/responsibility and the nation-state is the primary political unit, the OMC is a messy halfway house where Euro-bureaucrats go to exchange national policy platitudes and has little or no relevance to national policy developments. From a complexity perspective, OMC is a reasonable satisfying strategy for promoting learning and adaptational behaviour in a fundamentally oppositional environment. For example, if we return to our standard figure the relationship between the UK and EU employment policy systems would look something like that shown in Figure 5.1.

From this perspective it is easy to see that due to the fundamental distinctiveness between the member state and EU–UK employment policy systems, 'hard' linear policies demanding a radical convergence of these systems is extremely unlikely in the short term. Added to this divergence is the unwillingness of member states to give up national controls in the area of employment, reflected in the unanimous voting procedures within the Council for many aspects of employment policy. Hence, both at the level of the core short-term framework and EU institutions, substantial traditional policy developments (Regulations, Directives, etc) were clearly unlikely and most probably counterproductive. Hence, the 1990s saw the emergence of new methods, the OMC, for bypassing these fundamental blockages. The OMC operates at the emergent adaptational level of biotic and conscious complexity, focusing on

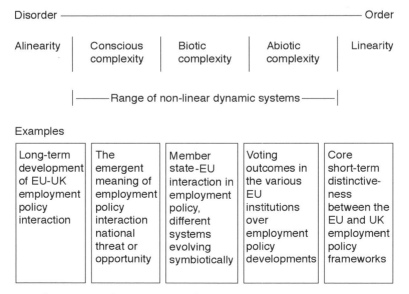

Figure 5.1 The range of EU–UK employment policy interaction.

encouraging symbiotic interaction and learning. This does not mean that it can overcome the fundamental distinctiveness of the different systems in the short term. However, it has the potential to shift the meaning of employment policy interaction from threat to opportunity and, over the long term, fundamentally shift the nature of the distinctiveness between the systems.

Complexity does not imply that the OMC was inevitable given the fundamental differences between the employment policy systems, or that OMC will automatically lead to a greater convergence. What it means is that it was not strange or surprising that an OMC-like strategy emerged in the 1990s to address the stalemate in employment policy, and that it is unlikely to alter the basic distinctiveness of the system in the short term. However, given that the fundamental boundaries of the EU–UK relationship remain in place (the UK doesn't leave the EU, the EU doesn't break apart, etc) OMC would have a tendency to lower the distinctiveness of the systems and eventually bring about some form of fundamental shift in their relationships. However, the exact nature of this fundamental shift quickly pushes us into the alinear 'box', and we are left projecting our hopes and guesses onto the eventual outcome.

Notes

[1] Especially the employment rate targets contained under Section A of the horizontal Guidelines and Guidelines 1–3 of the Employability Pillar.

[2] The Working Families' Tax Credit (WFTC) was introduced in April 2000 to provide extra assistance for working families with children and is estimated to deliver an average £30 extra a week to 1 million families. Further tax credits have also been developed in the form of the Disabled Person's Tax Credit (DPTC), and in April 2000 the Children's Tax Credit (CTC). Paid at a rate of £10 per week, this effectively provides a tax cut of up to £520 pounds a year for around 5 million families (DWP 2001).

[3] Reform of NICs is claimed to have taken an estimated 1 million low-paid workers out of the system while maintaining their benefit entitlements. The new 10p starting rate of income tax has also been introduced with the aim of benefiting those on low incomes (DWP 2001).

[4] The introduction of the national minimum wage is estimated to have raised the wages of an estimated 1.3 million low-paid workers by 15% (ECOTEC Research and Consulting 2002: 26).

[5] Figures for England show expenditure on education and training increased from £33 029 million in the period 1997–1998 to £38 204 in the period 2000–2001 (ECOTEC Research and Consulting 2002: 32).

Chapter 6

Europe leading the way? The EU as agenda setter in British equal opportunities policy

Despite the general weakness of European Union (EU) social policy, gender policy (or equal opportunities policy as it is called at the EU level) has been one of the few exceptions. During the 'first wave' of EU gender policy in the 1960s and 1970s, the European Commission, with a clear but narrow treaty base in Article 119,[1] emerged as a leading advocate of policies to promote sex equality within the workplace and statutory equality rights between men and women in terms of pay and treatment at work. The 'second wave' in the 1980s and early 1990s saw a significant expansion of the EU gender policy framework, growth of new gender policy actors and creation of a strong gender policy 'advocacy coalition' (Mazey 1998: 137). In recent years, the growing influence of gender policy actors, and their frustration with traditional policy tactics, prompted the EU to embrace innovative action initiatives and gender mainstreaming in what can be seen as a distinct 'third wave' of EU gender policy activism. As a result of these advances, equal opportunities policy is today widely regarded as the 'most highly developed pillar of the EC's social policy' (Barnard 2000a: 197).

Due to the relative weakness of UK gender policy, EU gender policy has played a significant role in the UK on a number of levels. The expansive rulings of the European Court on the 'first wave' gender directives served as a powerful force of vertical Europeanisation in Britain. In the area of labour policy, 'the impact of EC labour law on UK labour law has been greatest in the field of equality between the sexes' (Bercusson 1996: 29). The gender equalisation aspects of the structural funds have had a noticeable impact on UK female employment patterns. This influence is particularly impressive given the confrontational stance towards European sex equality laws from the 1979–1997 Conservative Government (Crawley and Slowey 1995; Nott 1999). In 1997, when the Labour Government signed the Social Chapter it ensured that British gender policy would continue to be heavily influenced by European legislation and litigation. This is particularly true given the development and success of gender mainstreaming strategies in the UK. Hence, because Britain had and still has amongst the weakest gender rights and entitlements of all member states, EU gender policy developments remain on the cutting edge of UK policy. In this sense, in many areas, the EU acts as more than just a policy floor, but even as an agenda setter for UK gender policy.

Equal opportunities: the 'first wave' of European regulation

The notion that the state is responsible for pursuing policies to promote equal opportunities between men and women is a relatively recent phenomenon. During the construction of Europe's welfare models in the post-war period, concepts of sex equality did not feature prominently in their overall design (Mazey 1998: 137). Within this traditional policy frame women were defined largely in terms of dependent wives and mothers. This conception was particularly strong in Britain compared, for example, to the countries of Scandinavia.

Although this traditional policy frame had remained largely static for generations, by the 1960s it was being challenged by a strong 'second-wave' feminist movement, campaigning for gender equality in both the public and private spheres (Crompton 1997). At the European level, when the EU was founded in 1957 the traditional 'male-breadwinner' policy frame was still dominant. As such there existed little understanding or appreciation among Europe's political leaders of the inequalities and discrimination encountered by women within the workplace. However, in Article 119, the treaty *did* provide an explicit and unambiguous commitment to the principle of equal pay between men and women:

> *Each Member State shall during the first stage ensure and subsequently maintain the application of the principle that men and women should receive equal pay for equal work.*

At the time, pay discrimination was the most visible and direct form of discrimination encountered by women, and a common practice in the post-war years. Article 119, though motivated more by fears of competition from cut-price female labour than a desire for gender equality (Hoskyns 1996), did provide the Commission with a solid, if narrow, legal basis upon which to construct European gender equality policy. Indeed, Mazey (1998: 142) argued that, 'it is the hook upon which all subsequent EC legislation in this sector hangs'.

Throughout the 1960s and 1970s, women's groups intensified their campaign for workplace equality within national policy-making arenas. Unsurprisingly, some elements of the women's movement focused their lobbying activity at the European level. With women comprising half the Community's population and evenly distributed in all member states, it is easy to understand why the European Parliament and Commission were willing to support the interests of this particular group of marginalised workers. Consequently, both the European Commission and Parliament responded by developing committees to represent women's interests. In this mutually beneficial relationship, women's groups were able to use the European policy in an attempt to win legal rights they could not gain domestically, while this emerging policy area also helped to legitimise the new European political system. The outcome of this heightened political activity was the adoption of a number of equality directives that constituted a 'first wave' of EC gender legislation, most importantly the Equal Pay Directive (EPD) and Equal Treatment Directive (Rees 1998).

Clarifying and expanding the scope of Article 119, the 1975 Equal Pay Directive (EPD) was the first European gender Directive to be adopted and was relatively uncontroversial given the explicit reference to the principle of equal pay in the Rome Treaty.[2] Article 1 of the Directive expanded the definition of equal pay to include 'the same work or for work to which equal value is attributed'. In Article 2, member states were required to introduce measures within their national legal systems to enable employees to seek judicial redress if they considered themselves to have been discriminated against. Article 6 demanded that effective means of enforcement were available.

In the following year the Equal Treatment Directive (ETD) extended earlier equal pay legislation.[3] Similarities in format and language revealed that the two Directives were intended to complement one another to create a solid foundation of legal rights to aid the fight against sex discrimination. Yet, whereas the EPD passed through the Community's legislative procedures with relative ease, the ETD underwent nine revisions before securing adoption (Geyer 2000a: 112). During this process, provisions relating to social security were withdrawn from the ambit of the Directive, while ambitious proposals concerning childcare, paternity leave and the burden of proof in sex discrimination cases were also excluded (Burrows and Mair 1996: 47; Geyer 2000a: 112). Article 1 of the final Directive proclaimed the purpose of the legislation was to:

> *put into effect in the Member States the principle of equal treatment for men and women as regards access to employment, including promotion, and to vocational training and as regards working conditions.*

While the Directives on equal pay and equal treatment were the most significant laws adopted during this 'first wave' of European policy activism, further related Directives were adopted in 1979 on equal treatment within statutory social security schemes,[4] and in 1986 on equal treatment in occupational social security schemes[5] and equal treatment of self-employed workers.[6] However, although the 1979 Directive caused some controversy amongst the member states, none of the Directives were particularly far-reaching. Given the relative weakness of the Commission and gender policy actors and the general policy stagnation at the time, it is surprising that there were any legislative developments at all.

Equal opportunities in Britain: the Equal Pay and Sex Discrimination Acts

Although heavily influenced by a traditional 'male-breadwinner' policy frame, the adoption of the 1970 Equal Pay Act (EPA) and the 1975 Sex Discrimination Act (SDA) briefly made Britain an international pioneer in advancing formal gender equality rights. Though emerging before the EPD and ETD, these Acts may have been influenced by European developments. Britain was joining the EU in 1975 and governmental elites would have been well aware of recent EU legislation. Moreover, the two Acts and Directives complemented each other so well that the UK did not initially introduce any further legislation to implement the two Directives (Mazey 1998: 47).

Following increased pressure from the women's movement and the trade unions for statutory equal opportunities policies, Labour's Minister for

Employment, Barbara Castle, successfully secured the passage of the Equal Pay Act in 1970. In its original form, the EPA gave individuals a right to the same contractual pay and benefits as a person of the opposite sex (EOC 2002a). The Sex Discrimination Act of 1975 was a broader piece of legislation that made discrimination on the grounds of sex or marital status unlawful in employment, training, education and the provision of goods and services. Under the Act, discrimination can either be direct or indirect. Direct discrimination refers to a situation where a woman (or a man) is treated less favourably than a person of the opposite sex in comparable circumstances, solely due to their sex. The more complex notion of indirect discrimination refers to situations where a condition or requirement is applied to both sexes, but:

- this adversely affects a considerably larger proportion of one sex than the other, and
- the condition or requirement cannot be justified by factors irrespective of sex (EOC 2002b).

Significantly, the SDA does not specify the tests to be applied in determining what is or is not justifiable, leaving this to be determined by the courts. Finally, the SDA also established the independent Equal Opportunities Commission (EOC) and awarded it a number of specific powers, including the right to provide legal advice and assistance to individuals in bringing sex discrimination claims, and powers to bring legal proceedings in the name of the EOC (EOC 2002c).

The two British Acts, like the European Directives that followed, conceived the issue of equality through an equal rights/equal treatment framework. By providing 'individualistic' and 'protective' rights, the underlying assumption of this legislative approach was that 'the prevailing system is essentially a fair one, although there may be isolated cases where a particular individual is treated unfairly' (Bagilhole 1997: 92). To remedy these instances, an appropriate policy response is one that confers upon women the same rights that are enjoyed by men. Despite the similar foundations underpinning the British and European legislation, concerns were soon raised as to how adequately the EPA and SDA implemented the provisions of the two main European gender Directives (Beveridge *et al.* 2000b: 177).

The influence of the European Court of Justice

At first, the directives on equal pay and equal treatment had little impact on UK legal developments, particularly after the 1979 Conservative election victory (Alter and Vargas 2000: 455). However, during the 1980s and 1990s successive rulings from the European Court of Justice (ECJ) clarified and extended the scope of Article 119 and the gender directives (Mazey 1998: 147). By the early 1990s, the ECJ was generally acknowledged as one of the most powerful and influential institutional actors in gender policy.

The ECJ cannot initiate proceedings itself; its ability to issue rulings is dependent on cases being referred to it for judgement. For equal opportunities cases, referrals to the Court have been launched from two main sources. Under Article 169 of the Rome Treaty, the Commission can initiate infringement proceedings within the ECJ against member states that are deemed to have responded inadequately to their legal Community obligations. Alternatively, under Article 177 national courts may refer cases to the ECJ, either for points of clarification or to resolve questions of incompatibility between Community and national law (Bainbridge 1998: 105–106). In both instances the significance of ECJ rulings rests upon the doctrine of supremacy of EU law over national law.

For example, in 1980 the Commission commenced infringement proceedings against the UK Government under Article 169 for inadequate implementation of the EPD. The Commission argued that the EPA failed to ensure the principle of equal pay for work of equal value. Although the EPA made provision for job evaluation schemes, the UK legislation did not permit the introduction of these schemes without the employer's prior consent. The Commission highlighted that where this was refused by the employer, the Act failed to provide any alternative means of determining whether work could be considered of equal value for pay purposes (Craig and de Burca 1995: 798). In supporting the Commission's argument the ECJ ruled:

> *The UK's interpretation amounts to a denial of the very existence of a right to equal pay for work of equal value where no classification has been made* (Case 61/81, *Commission* v. *United Kingdom*).[7]

Although the Conservative Government strongly disagreed with the ruling, it was compelled to amend the EPA accordingly, which it did through the Equal Pay (Amendment) Regulations 1983. The Regulations introduced a third test of 'equal value' into equal pay cases. This has since been used to determine whether two different jobs place equal demands on workers in terms of effort, skill and decision making (Bagilhole 1997: 73). As a result of these new procedures, the House of Lords in *Hayward* v. *Cammell Laird*[8] upheld the claim of a female cook that her work was of equal value with that of male painters, thermal insulation engineers and joiners working for the same employer.

In a second Article 169 referral to the ECJ, the Commission alleged that by limiting access to training for male midwives, the SDA contravened Article 2 of the ETD. In Case 165/82 *Commission* v. *United Kingdom*, the ECJ rejected the Commission's argument by accepting that 'personal sensitivities' could have a significant impact on the relationship between midwife and patient (Craig and de Burca 1995: 838). The constraints placed upon male midwives in the UK were deemed justifiable under the terms of the ETD. Nevertheless, in a further complaint raised in the same case, the ECJ ruled that by excluding private households and firms with five or fewer workers from the provisions of the Act, the SDA *was* in breach of the ETD. As a result the Conservative Government was forced to amend the SDA in 1986 to extend the Act's provisions to these excluded categories of workers.

In both cases, ECJ rulings forced a reluctant Conservative Government to significantly alter its legislation. However, there are obvious limits to the ECJ rulings in the UK. For example, in the case of the amendments to the equal pay legislation, the new procedures were seen to be 'so burdensome and unnecessarily complicated ... that many suspected the Government of sabotaging the original equal pay legislation for which it had never held sympathy' (in Alter and Vargas 2000: 457).

Despite this, the ECJ has had an even greater impact on equal opportunities rights in Britain through its rulings in the large number of cases referred from the national courts via the Article 177 procedure (Gold 1993: 8). Many of these referrals were the result of sustained litigation strategies launched by various equal opportunities actors across Europe – most notably by the Equal Opportunities Commission in Britain. As a result of these cases the Court has issued a series of rulings that have extended the scope and protections afforded by Article 119 and the early gender directives. With various policy actors willing to use European litigation and the Court prepared to deliver expansive rulings on the boundaries of Europe's equality laws, both the Government and private employers have been shown that non-compliance with Community legislation could prove costly in both financial and political terms (Alter and Vargas 2000: 462–3).

The successful use of EU law litigation strategies to extend gender rights is unparalleled by any other social policy sector and due to a convergence of distinctive factors (Barnard 1994; Alter and Vargas 2000). First, a strong body of EU law must exist that potential litigants can draw upon in the national courts. By granting Article 119 and later the ETD *direct* effect,[9] the Court ruled that these legal instruments gave rise to legal rights which individuals could have enforced directly within national courts without the need for further national implementing legislation. Second, domestic policy actors must be willing to use European litigation to achieve their objectives. In Britain, individual lawyers, the EOC and the TUC have actively pursued a European litigation strategy. Third, since private litigants must rely on the national judiciary to make referrals to the ECJ, support within the national courts is essential. During the 1980s the majority of British courts were keen to minimise the involvement of the ECJ in the British legal system. However, the EOC successfully found support for its actions amongst a number of industrial tribunals. Even though industrial tribunals represented 'the lowest rung of the judicial hierarchy' (Alter and Vargas 2000: 460), the fact that any judge, at any level, anywhere in the Community can make an Article 177 referral to the ECJ meant this particular avenue was enough.

As a result of these factors, gender equality actors have managed to win a number of important legal victories including: the definition of pay, concept of indirect discrimination, notably in relation to part-time workers, rights of pregnant workers and the equalisation of the state pensionable age in the UK. Details of key cases and their impacts are found in Box 6.1.

Box 6.1 Key cases and their impacts

Extending the definition of pay

In a series of rulings the Court established that 'pay', as defined by Article 119 and the EPD, covers a wide range of payments. These rulings have enabled British and European workers to claim equal pay in respect of *ex gratia* payments made following the end of employment, established in *Garland;*[a] statutory sick pay in *Rinner-Kühn;*[b] and redundancy payments and payments made under a private occupational pension scheme, established in the EOC-backed *Barber* case.[c]

Developing the concept of indirect discrimination

In *Jenkins*,[d] later clarified and extended in *Bilka*,[e] *Enderby*[f] and *Rinner-Kühn*,[g] the Court ruled that paying part-time workers less than their full-time counterparts contravened European equal pay laws, if the difference in pay rates could not be objectively justified by factors other than the workers' sex (EOC 2001). As women account for 90% of all part-time workers in the Community, this had an obvious gender impact.

Developing the rights of pregnant workers

In *Dekker*,[h] the ECJ ruled that a refusal to employ a candidate on grounds of pregnancy constituted direct discrimination, while in *Hertz*,[i] it concluded that dismissal due to pregnancy also amounted to direct discrimination. Later, in *Webb*,[j] the Court firmly rejected the comparison of a pregnant worker with a sick man to determine whether a dismissal constituted discrimination. This judgement overturned a number of earlier rulings by the British courts on the scope of the Sex Discrimination Act.

Equalisation of state pensionable age

The *Marshall* case had significant implications for equalising the retirement ages for men and women in Britain.[k] Ms Marshall, a local health authority worker, was dismissed after having passed the compulsory retirement age of 60 (the state pensionable age for women) while her male counterparts were required to retire at 65. The European Court concluded that this was discriminatory, and although the judgement did not formally require Britain to align the state pensionable age for men and women, the ruling along with others convinced the Government to level up the normal pensionable age for both sexes to 65 (Burrows and Mair 1996: 96).[l]

[a] Case 12/81 *Garland* v. *British Rail Engineering Ltd* (1982).
[b] Case 171/88 *Rinner-Kühn* v. *FWW Spezial-Gebäudereinigung GmbH* (1989).
[c] Case C–262/88 *Barber* v. *Guardian Royal Exchange* (1990).
[d] Case 96/80 *Jenkins* v. *Kingsgate (Clothing Productions Ltd)* (1981).
[e] Case 170/84 *Bilka-Kaufhaus GmbH* v. *Karin Weber von Hartz* (1986).
[f] Case 127/92 *Enderby* v. *Frenchay Health Authority and the Secretary of State for Health* (1994).
[g] Case 171/88 *Rinner-Kühn*.
[h] Case C–177/88 *Dekker* v. *Stichting Voringscentrum voor Jonge Volwassenen Plus* (1990).
[i] Case C-179/88 *Handels-og Kontorfunktionærernes Forbund i Danmark* v. *Dansk Arbejdsgiverforening* (1990).
[j] Case C-32/93 *Webb* v. *EMO Air Cargo (UK) Ltd* (1994).
[k] Case 152/84 *Marshall* v. *Southampton and South West Hants Area Health Authority* (1986).
[l] These changes were made through the Pension Act 1995.

Clearly, from the early 1980s to the present day, the jurisprudence of the ECJ has been extremely influential in extending the scope of the EU's early equality directives and as Lord Lester, an early gender equality campaigner argued, it has also 'enabled the EOC and individual women and men to win in the courts what we in the mid-1970s could not win in Whitehall and Westminster' (Mazey 1998: 147).

Not surprisingly, despite these changes criticisms of Britain's equal opportunities laws persists. Both the EOC and Trades Union Congress (TUC) have consistently argued that the EPA and SDA fail to fully address the true extent of discrimination encountered by British women. Describing the current EPA as a 'paradise for lawyers, but hell for women' (Bagilhole 1997: 94), the EOC has actively campaigned for the Government to reform the existing legal framework and take account of the continuing gender pay gap – the largest pay gap within the EU (European Industrial Relations Observatory (EIRO), April 2001f). In May 2001 the Labour Government responded to these criticisms by announcing a package of measures to make the existing legislation 'simpler, faster and fairer' (EIRO, March 2001d). However, to date, it rejected a major reform of the much-maligned SDA.

Broader developments: the 'second wave' of European equality law

In the 1990s, following the general revival of European integration and the success of the Social Charter, Europe's gender policy actors began pushing for a 'second wave' of equality Directives. Using a new 'policy frame' where equality is conceptualised in terms of the need to promote an 'equality of outcome' (Mazey 2001: 7) and policies should enable 'men and women to reconcile their occupational and family obligations' (European Commission 1990: Point 16), the EU developed and passed four new Directives that sought to establish minimum requirements for the treatment of pregnant workers, provision of parental leave, rights of part-time workers and rights of workers on fixed-term contracts. As we shall see, though primarily confirming existing 'best practice' and loosely implemented at the national level, these Directives have had a significant impact on the British gender policy regime.

The Pregnancy Directive

As discussed earlier, the ECJ had considered the issue of pregnancy under the provisions of the ETD and conferred a number of rights on pregnant women in the workplace. In the 1989 SAP, the Commission expressed its desire to strengthen these rights by introducing a Directive to establish minimum standards of protection for pregnant workers. In October 1992 the Community responded by adopting Council Directive 92/85/EEC – 'The Pregnancy Directive'. This was the first gender Directive to break from the earlier 'equal treatment' framework by accepting that pregnancy represents a fundamental difference between men and women.

Based on Article 118a, the Pregnancy Directive was justified primarily in terms of promoting improvements in the safety and health at work of pregnant workers and workers who have recently given birth or are breast-feeding (Blanpain and Engels 1998: 298). However, by establishing minimum standards for the provision of maternity leave, the Directive also contained strong social objectives, such as seeking to help mothers maintain their attachment to the labour market while fulfilling their parental responsibilities (Hatt 1997: 157). As the Commission argued in a 1999 implementation report, 'The rights set out in the Directive represent a good framework for the dual role of women as workers and as mothers, roles which require both special protection and non-discrimination' (European Commission 1999a: 22). For these reasons, it was opposed by the British Conservative Government but passed through the EU Council due to the qualified majority voting (QMV) procedures for health and safety issues. No further legal challenge was mounted.

The Pregnancy Directive establishes minimum standards for the treatment of pregnant workers. The main provisions include:

- workplace risk assessment
- risk avoidance
- restrictions on night work for pregnant women and new mothers
- maternity leave
- rights against dismissal
- 'adequate' maternity leave allowances.

Overall, the Directive established a number of basic rights, but these were generally below the member state average. As Ellis concluded, 'the directive will require little or no change to the law in any Member State apart from the UK' (in Bercusson 1996: 29).

The Parental Leave Directive

The Commission first proposed a Directive on parental leave in 1983. This would have allowed either parent to take three months' parental leave up to the child's third birthday, and an unspecified number of days off work for 'family reasons'. With no existing statutory provision for parental leave in the UK, this proposal was strongly opposed by the deregulatory-minded Conservative Government. Indeed, the British veto was used to prevent the unanimous approval necessary for the draft Directive's adoption. A decade later, the Belgian Council Presidency revived the issue with a new draft directive. Again, these entitlements to parental leave for both men and women were designed to enable workers to reconcile work and family commitments, while also attempting to overcome the notion of women as primary carers. However, with negotiations again unable to overcome British opposition, the Commission decided by Autumn 1994 to defer responsibility for negotiations to the Social Partners, in accordance with the Maastricht Social Policy Agreement (Falkner 1998).

As the cross-industry organisations the Union des Industries de la Communauté Européene (UNICE), CEEP and the European Trade Union Confederation (ETUC) began talks, hopes of a successful conclusion were high. The issue was perceived to be relatively uncontroversial, while the Confederation of British Industry (CBI) was only invited to the negotiations as an observer with no right of veto. This optimism was vindicated when the Social Partners informed the Commission that they had successfully concluded the first framework agreement under the new Maastricht procedures. This agreement was made legally binding by the adoption of a Council Directive in June 1996.[10] In accordance with the principle of subsidiarity, the agreement contained only a few modest stipulations to:

- create minimum requirements for reconciling work and family life, including a right to three months' unpaid maternity leave
- encourage employers and employees to determine their own workplace agreements on parental leave
- require member states, in the absence of workplace agreements, to set minimum provisions in the form, duration and circumstances of parental leave.

The main provisions for parental leave were thus left to be determined either directly by the member states, or through negotiated agreements between management and labour. When the Labour Government signed the Social Chapter in 1997, the existing provisions of the Parental Leave Directive were extended to Britain.

The Directives on part-time and fixed-term work

Although the issue of flexible contracts does not relate directly to gender equality, 'atypical' or 'non-standard' forms of employment have significant indirect implications. During the 1980s and 1990s the incidence of flexible working practices, such as part-time and fixed-term work, became increasingly common. Significantly, women occupied the majority of these positions. On the one hand, flexible work of this nature was seen to offer advantages to both working parents and businesses. Individuals could arrange their working time to serve both their occupational and family obligations, while employers could align working patterns more closely with the needs of production or output. On the other hand, these atypical forms of employment also left the predominantly female workforce particularly vulnerable, often lacking the statutory protections of their mainstream counterparts. The sex discrimination legislation of the 1970s aimed to award women the same legal rights as a 'typical' (full-time and permanent) male worker (Burrows and Mair 1996: 133). Although the rulings of the ECJ had provided some recognition of women's rights as part-time workers (Hantrais 2002: 119), by 1989 the Commission felt European legislation was needed to protect the rights of atypical workers while promoting the development of this mutually beneficial form of employment.

After a number of legislative proposals on atypical work were blocked in the Council during the early 1990s, the Commission announced in 1994 that it would defer responsibility for concluding a framework agreement to the Social Partners. The successful outcome of these negotiations culminated in the adoption of the 1997 Council Directive on part-time work.[11] This was soon followed by the adoption of the Council Directive on fixed-term work in 1999.[12] Again, both frameworks agreements proceeded with a light regulatory approach (Kenner 1999: 42) and included provisions to:

- ensure that part-time and fixed-term workers are not treated less favourably than comparable full-time or permanent workers
- 'facilitate the development of part-time work on a voluntary basis'
- prevent abuse arising from the use of successive fixed-term contracts.

Implementing the 'second wave' in the UK: the 'family-friendly' agenda

With the exception of the 1992 Pregnancy Directive, implementation of the 'second wave' of European gender directives fell upon Tony Blair's Labour Government. Whereas the Conservative's implementation of the Pregnancy Directive was undertaken in a reluctant manner characteristic of the party's attitude to the 'first wave' of gender Directives, Labour came to office proclaiming a strong commitment to developing a 'family-friendly' employment agenda. The 1998 White Paper: *Fairness at Work* acknowledged that 'work and parenthood can create conflicting pressures' (DTI 1998: 5.1). With women expected to account for 75% of the increase in the UK labour force over the next 10 years, Labour argued that businesses need to make greater efforts to promote family-friendly employment practices (EIRO 1999h) and that 'helping employees to combine work and family life satisfactorily is good not only for parents and children but also for businesses' (DTI 1998: 5.1). To give substance to this agenda, Labour introduced a number of independent legislative changes such as the national minimum wage, Working Families' Tax Credits and the 2002 Employment Act that gives parents of children under the age of six the right to request flexible working arrangements (EIRO 2001a). With the exception of these nationally inspired initiatives, the majority of the proposals contained under Labour's 'family-friendly' employment agenda were directly linked to European gender Directives.

However, in spite of Labour's decision to sign the Social Chapter, and its public commitment to reconciling work and family life, the new Government's initial transposition of these 'second wave' Directives was undertaken in a minimalist manner not dissimilar to its Conservative predecessor (McKay 2001: 291–7). While Britain was obliged to introduce new statutory entitlements in relation to parental leave, part-time work and fixed-term contracts, Labour initially sought to exploit the full flexibility provided by these directives, reflecting both political and economic concerns about the cost of mounting 'red tape' on British companies (EIRO, February 2001g: 3). During the consultation period prior to the implementation of the regulations, business groups were extremely active in lobbying the Labour Government. Consequently, although the Directives demanded the introduction or extension of a range of statutory rights, the flexibility of the 'second wave' gender Directives enabled the Government to establish a relatively low level of minimum entitlements. Later, under pressure from domestic critics, Labour did make a number of improvements in some entitlements. Overall, in this area, the EU was an initiator of policy developments, but its impact has been limited by both Conservative and Labour governmental resistance.

Implementing the Pregnancy Directive

Formally a health and safety law, the Pregnancy Directive places an important obligation on employers to undertake risk assessments in relation to pregnant employees and those who have recently given birth. However, for Britain, the most significant requirements arising from the Directive relate to the provisions on maternity leave and maternity pay. The UK first introduced a system of statutory maternity leave in 1976. In offering a maximum of 40 weeks' maternity leave, Britain's provisions appeared to be very generous. Yet as Sue Hatt (1997: 158) exclaimed, 'appearances however can be misleading!' To be eligible for this period of leave, a woman had to have been continuously employed at her place of work for at least two years. Figures for 1988 showed this effectively excluded 40% of women from claiming any maternity leave. Complying with the 1992 Directive therefore required Britain to significantly amend its existing legislation (Bercusson 1996: 29).

In response to the Article 8 requirement for a 'continuous period of maternity leave of at least 14 weeks', the Conservative Government introduced a new right to *ordinary* maternity leave for all female employees irrespective of hours of work or continuity of employment (Burrows and Mair 1996: 165).[13] Although this represents a marked improvement in the coverage of women eligible for maternity leave, by providing the minimum period of 14 weeks permitted by the Directive, the UK provisions were the least generous in the EU and compared unfavourably with the 28 weeks' leave granted to women employed in Denmark (European Commission 1999a: 10–11). The Directive also required that workers on maternity leave must be provided with an 'adequate allowance'. It limits the use of eligibility conditions to a period of prior employment not in excess of 12 months. As a result, the Government was forced to amend Britain's systems of Statutory Maternity Pay (SMP) and Maternity Allowance (MA). Following the 1994 amendments, women were eligible for SMP if they had been continuously employed for 26 weeks at the qualifying week, and received average earnings in the previous eight weeks above the threshold for National Insurance Contributions (NICs). Where a woman met these conditions she was entitled to SMP for a total of 18 weeks. During the first six weeks she was entitled to 90% of her average weekly pay and for the remaining 13 weeks to a weekly payment of £52.50. Although this represented a marked improvement on the previous system, it did lead to the anomalous situation whereby many women were legally entitled to 18 weeks' maternity pay, but eligible for only 14 weeks' *ordinary* leave. For some women not eligible for SMP, further financial assistance was provided through the payment of Maternity Allowance (MA). MA could be claimed by women who have paid NICs in respect of at least 26 weeks out of the 66 weeks preceding the expected week of childbirth.

Although the Conservative's 1994 Regulations appeared to comply with the terms of the Directive, many commentators were highly critical of their complexity and the minimal entitlements they provided. Some argued that the limited financial assistance granted by SMP and MA forced many women who wished, or needed, to return to work after childbirth, to do so before the end of their statutory leave entitlement. Others noted that the Regulations effectively excluded 'some of the poorest women with children' who were most in need of a system of statutory maternity pay (Burrows and Mair 1996: 168). Following Labour's election in 1997, the new Government has voluntarily overseen a significant improvement in the provisions for maternity leave and maternity pay through the 1999 Employment Relations Act and 2002 Employment Act 2002 (DTI 2000).

The 1999 Act increased the period of *ordinary* maternity leave for all employees to 18 weeks (up from 14 weeks), benefiting a further 85 000 women, and reduced the eligibility requirements for *additional* maternity leave to one year's employment (McColgan 2000a: 129; Tucker 2000: 80). The 2002 Act created new maternity leave provisions for women who were expecting to give birth on or after 6 April 2003. The length of *ordinary* maternity leave was increased to 26 weeks' leave. *Additional* maternity leave will begin immediately after ordinary maternity leave and continue for a further 26 weeks, while the qualification period for additional maternity leave was reduced to 26 weeks' continuous employment. Regarding maternity pay, the 1999 changes also extended SMP and MA to cover the whole of the *ordinary* maternity leave period of 18 weeks, thereby ending the anomaly within the Conservatives' Regulations. Also, the 2002 changes extended the period covered by SMP and MA and increased the amount paid. Summarising the outcome of this complex series of change, the EOC has noted that from April 2003 most mothers will be entitled to six months' paid and six months' unpaid maternity leave (EOC 2002d: 2), a significant increase over earlier entitlements.

Implementing the Parental Leave Directive

Given that Britain had previously provided no statutory entitlement to family-related leave, implementing the 1996 Parental Leave Directive represented a radical departure for UK employment law (McColgan 2000a: 134). The Labour Government transposed the Directive through the 1999 Maternity and Parental Leave Regulations and 1999 Employment Relations Act.

Despite these Acts and a number of amendments, the Government's implementation was widely regarded as a minimalist interpretation of the Directive's provisions. For example, the original 1999 Regulations provided working parents in the UK with a statutory right to 13 weeks' unpaid leave to be taken up to the child's fifth birthday, where the child was born on or after 15 December 1999. This constituted the minimum period of leave permitted by the Directive and excluded all parents before the December start. Similarly, reflecting the Directive's preference for parental leave arrangements to be determined by management and labour, the Regulations encourage employers and employees to conclude either: collective agreements with trade unions, 'workforce agreements' with elected representatives, or individual agreements. In the absence of a negotiated agreement, the Regulations contain a 'fallback' scheme. This determines the *minimum entitlements* for how parental leave may be taken. In formulating these provisions the Labour Government again sought to exploit the full flexibility afforded by the Directive. The fallback scheme states that:

- leave must be taken in blocks or multiples of one week with a limit of four weeks leave in a year
- 21 days' notice must be given

- an employer may postpone leave for up to 6 months where business cannot cope, although leave cannot be postponed when the employee has given notice to take leave immediately after the time the child is born.

The 1999 Employment Relations Act established the legal right for employees to take time off for urgent family reasons. Again management and labour were given considerable scope to determine how this right was to be exercised. The Act merely required that employees possess the right to take 'a reasonable amount of time off' to 'take action which is necessary' in the event of illness, injury, death of a dependant, or where care arrangements break down. No statutory limits were established to determine the length of time that may be deemed 'reasonable'.

Responding to the 1999 Regulations, the CBI accepted they represented 'a reasonable balance between individual rights and business needs' (EIRO 1999a). Britain's business leaders were particularly satisfied that the Government bowed to their demands that parental leave should apply up to the child's fifth rather than eighth birthday, and only in respect of children born after the Directive's implementation date (EIRO 1999h). Although the TUC welcomed the Regulations as a 'historic milestone on the road to making work family-friendly', they were concerned that because parental leave in the UK was to be unpaid, few would be willing to take it and it would punish the working poor who needed it the most. UK and European research clearly indicated that parental leave uptake depends on whether it is paid or unpaid (EIRO 1999g; McColgan 2000a). A second criticism concerned the Government's decision to restrict the leave entitlement to parents of children born on or after 15 December 1999 – the date the Regulations took effect. As the Directive made no provision for member states to introduce such criteria, the TUC argued that this restriction was unlawful. With 2.7 million parents consequently excluded from the statutory right to parental leave, the TUC opted to challenge the legality of this provision. In May 2000 the High Court referred the matter to the ECJ for a definitive ruling.

In response to these complaints, the Government introduced a number of amendments to the 1999 Regulations. The Employment Act 2002 entitles male employees whose children are born on or after 6 April 2003 to two weeks' paid paternity leave in addition to the existing right to 13 weeks' parental leave (EIRO 2002e). Statutory Paternity Pay (SPP) will be paid at the same standard rate as SMP. The Act further states that in principle this leave is to be taken in one block within the first eight weeks after the child's birth (DTI 2002a). Again, this level of pay compares unfavourably with the entitlements elsewhere in the Union. In Sweden, fathers receive between 70% and 80% of their salary (McColgan 2000a: 140). In 2001 the Government introduced amendment Regulations to extend the right to parental leave to parents of children who were under five on 15 December 1999. This followed the European Commission's decision in April 2001 to issue the UK Government with a 'reasoned opinion', which argued the restriction contravened the Parental Leave Directive. Although the Government could have waited for the ECJ to deliver its definitive ruling, the fact that Britain appeared destined to lose the case – a similar judgement had already gone against the Irish – convinced the Government to voluntarily back down on this matter and introduce the necessary changes (EIRO, June 2000e; EIRO, May 2001g).

Implementing the Directives on part-time and fixed-term workers

In Britain today, one in four jobs are part-time. Women form a disproportionate number of part-time workers with 44% of all female employees working on a part-time basis compared to just 12% of male workers (Labour Market Trends, June 2000, in McKay 2001: 294). Meanwhile, the 1998 Workplace Industrial Relations Survey (WIRS) showed that 35% of British workplaces employed workers on a temporary basis or a fixed-term contract for less than one year (Milward *et al.* 1998). This amounts to between 1.1 and 1.3 million workers, with women, again, forming the majority (EIRO 2001b). In this context the adoption of the EU Directives on part-time work and fixed-term contracts potentially held great significance for the development of workplace equality in Britain. However, the Labour Government's implementation of these Directives has been widely condemned by social policy advocates, for offering limited protections to only a small proportion of these workers.

At the heart of the Part-Time Workers' Regulations 2000 is the apparently explicit provision that, 'A part-time worker has the right not to be treated less favourably by his [*sic*] employer than the employer treats a comparable full-time worker' (Regulation 5). Yet these new statutory rights for part-time workers rely on the existence of a full-time 'comparable worker' (EIRO 2000c). It is this requirement that diminishes the effectiveness of the new equality laws for the majority of British part-timers. A valid comparator must be: employed by the same employer and at the same establishment; employed under the same type of contract; and engaged in broadly similar work to the part-time worker. These conditions rule out the possibility of a hypothetical comparator, even though such a provision already exists in relation to claims under the Sex Discrimination Act. As many part-time workers are employed in grades or sectors with no comparable full-time worker, the Government's own estimates suggest that only one million of the UK's six million part-timers would be able to provide such a comparator. Furthermore, the Government's Regulatory Impact Assessment study has estimated that of these workers only 400 000 – fewer than 7% of all part-time workers – would benefit directly from the Regulations through increases in pay or non-wage benefits (McColgan 2000b: 263). Again, the reason for Labour's 'light touch' towards implementing the Regulations reflects the Government's desire for business support while complying with the European Directives (McKay 2001: 295).

Labour only recently implemented the 1999 Directive on fixed-term work through the 2002 Fixed-term Employees' Regulations. Although the transposition process should have been completed by 10 July 2001, the Government exploited the Directive's provision that allowed member states to postpone implementation for up to one year to take account of 'special difficulties' (EIRO 2001b). The Regulations state that fixed-term employees should not be treated less favourably than comparable permanent employees because they are employed on a fixed-term contract, unless this can be objectively justified. Furthermore, the Regulations limit the use of successive fixed-term contracts to four years unless the use of further fixed-term contracts can, again, be justified on objective grounds. Previously, the UK and Ireland had been the only member state not to provide statutory limits on either the number of contract renewals permitted, or the maximum duration of fixed-term contracts (EIRO 1999e: 4).

The recent adoption of the Fixed-term Employees' Regulations has also prompted the Government to amend the earlier regulations for part-time workers. Under the Fixed-term Employees Regulations, employees on a fixed-term contract may compare themselves with a colleague working on either a part-time or full-time basis. As such, the Government has argued that it 'seemed sensible' to amend the Part-time Workers' Regulations to allow individual part-timers from 1 October 2002, 'to compare themselves to a full-time colleague irrespective of whether either party's contract is permanent or fixed-term' (DTI 2002b). These changes have improved the position for part-time workers who previously had no full-time comparator, thereby addressing some of the earlier criticisms of the Part-time Workers' Regulations. Once again, this illustrates the Government's cautious approach towards introducing incremental improvements to the original implementing Regulations. Although these changes were prompted by the adoption of regulations to implement the Fixed-term Work Directive, they were introduced voluntarily and not as a result of any direct EU legislative demands.

EU action initiatives, gender mainstreaming and their impact on the UK

Despite a number of advancements, women in Britain and the rest of Europe continue to suffer from discrimination and inequality. British women continue to earn considerably less than their male counterparts, remain segregated in the lowest grade employment and experience lower participation rates (Nott 1999; Lönnroth 2002). In this context, gender policy actors came to accept that while statutory regulation has extended the formal rights afforded to many women, the law alone was unlikely to overcome the full range of inequalities that women encounter. Hence, a new strategy was needed, a 'positive action' strategy.

As early as the 1980s the EU began to develop a body of non-binding *action initiatives* on behalf of women. As the Framework Strategy on Gender Equality (2001–2005) explained, the EU's equal opportunities strategy comprises an integrated 'dual-track' approach. The first strand was premised on the notion that 'persistent inequalities continue to require the implementation of specific action in favour of women' (European Commission 2000b: 3). Although these 'reactive interventions' continued to take the form of 'hard laws' where appropriate, in recent years a range of soft-regulatory actions have been favoured, including a series of Community-funded Action Programmes, a host of specific Resolutions, Recommendations and Communications, and the inclusion of an equal opportunities 'pillar' in the European Employment Strategy. The second strand of the strategy endorsed the 'gender mainstreaming' approach. As discussed earlier, mainstreaming is a key tactic for going beyond the limits of a purely legislative strategy (Rees 2002). Although the direct impact of these soft forms of regulation on UK gender policy has been limited, they *have* enabled the EU to extend and consolidate its influence in other policy areas associated with the pursuit of gender equality.

In 1981 the Commission proposed the first of what has become a series of Equal Opportunities Action Programmes to 'promote the achievement of equal opportunities in practice' (Council of the European Communities 1982). These early programmes were influential in overseeing the institutionalisation of this policy sector at the European level (Mazey 1998: 145) and were fundamental to the creation and development of various European 'policy networks' and the influential European Women's Lobby (EWL). Furthermore, the Action Programmes subsidised a range of projects with a gender dimension (Roelofs 1995: 130). For example, the current Fifth Action Programme 2001–2005 focuses its financial resources on an annual 'priority theme' such as the gender pay gap or reconciliation of work and family life (European Commission 2002b: 11). Related to this are the ESF gender programmes, most significantly the New Opportunities for Women (NOW) initiative introduced in November 1990 with a budget of 156 million European Currency Units (ECUs) to assist the integration of women into the labour market and encourage them to start their own company, provide start-up subsidies and promote vocational training (Roelofs 1995: 137). Likewise, the Community's EQUAL initiative, with an overall budget of EUR 3 billion over six years, explores ways of combating inequality in employment (European Commission 2002c: 11). Through these programmes and funding initiatives, EU gender actors have been able to broaden the scope of the EU's gender policy agenda (Mazey 1998: 144).

While the Action Programmes have been used to advance the gender Directives discussed above, they have also promoted the development of a body of non-binding 'soft law'. Two prominent areas that have benefited from the adoption of these soft-forms of regulation are the protection of workers from sexual harassment and the provision of childcare. Following the publication of a 1987 Commission report, the Council passed a non-binding Resolution on the protection of the dignity of women and men at work that concluded that 'sexual harassment is a serious problem for many working women in the European Community', and that any 'unwanted, unreasonable or offensive' conduct of a sexual nature 'constitutes an intolerable violation of the dignity of workers' (Council of the European Communities 1990). Furthermore, in the wake of the Third Action Programme (1991–1995), the Commission was prompted to issue a Recommendation and a Code of Conduct[14] on measures to combat sexual harassment.[15] Regarding the provision of childcare, responding to the need identified in the 1989 Social Charter and the Third Action Programme for further measures to reconcile occupational and family obligations, the Council also passed a Recommendation on childcare in 1992.[16]

In both cases, 'soft' regulatory strategies were used in an attempt to achieve through persuasion what could not be achieved through regulatory coercion. Indeed, strong national opposition to a 1986 draft Directive on sexual harassment[17] prompted the Commission to turn to soft law, whereas significant differences in existing national practice precluded the pursuit of a Council Directive on childcare. Another example can be found in the attempts to push EU gender policy beyond the boundaries of the workplace through a Council Resolution on the state of women's health and combating domestic violence.[18]

In general, the direct impact of these Action Programmes and soft laws on the development of UK gender policy has been limited. However, their indirect and long-term significance should not be underestimated. In a number of instances the Commission has been able to use indirect policy approaches to open up a particular area for Community involvement (Cram 1997). Following the 'soft law' developments on sexual harassment during the early 1990s, the Council adopted a Directive to amend the 1976 Equal Treatment Directive in September 2002. This demonstrates that in certain instances soft laws can, ultimately, lead to binding European legislation. Furthermore, whilst the 1992 Recommendation on Childcare was instrumental in the subsequent adoption of the Parental Leave Directive (Szyszczak 2000a: 101), it has also been credited with ensuring childcare has featured prominently under the European Employment Strategy.

Since the 1997 Luxembourg Summit, the issue of gender equality has also benefited significantly from the inclusion of an equal opportunities 'pillar' in the European Employment Strategy (EES). In addition to raising the provision of affordable and accessible childcare, which forms part of the Community's broader agenda to reconcile work and family life, the pillar also calls upon the member states (and Social Partners) to introduce *positive* measures to tackle existing gender gaps. In this way, many of the Community's long-standing equal opportunities objectives are now being pursued through the 'Luxembourg Process' of the EES. Since 1999 the member states have also been required to adopt a gender mainstreaming approach in implementing the Guidelines across all four pillars. Meanwhile, under the 'horizontal objectives' of the EES, the member states have been asked to consider setting national targets for raising the rate of employment for women to 57% by January 2005 and 60% by 2010. As seen elsewhere, these are having a noticeable impact on the UK.

Despite these developments, EU gender policy activists have increasingly highlighted the limitations of the existing equality framework, criticising the equal treatment approach for establishing male behaviour patterns as the norm against which women are measured, thereby failing to address the root causes of inequality (Rees 1998). Similarly, the use of 'positive action' under the equality of opportunity approach was criticised for generating isolated policy acts, 'resorted to only when governments need to address a particular problem' (Nott 1999: 205). Furthermore, both these approaches have overwhelmingly focused on securing equality within the workplace, leaving the private sphere of the home and family largely untouched (Nott 1999: 204; Beveridge *et al.* 2000c: 385–6).

Gender mainstreaming seeks to overcome these weaknesses. In contrast to the equal treatment and equality of opportunity frameworks, gender mainstreaming was founded 'upon a recognition of gender differences between men and women in terms of their socio-economic status and family responsibilities' (Mazey 2001: 7–8). Thus rather than implementing specific measures to help women overcome instances of discrimination or inequality, mainstreaming involves incorporating a gender perspective into *all* areas of public policy. It is therefore a long-term strategy designed to take account of the possible effect of all policies and programmes on the respective situations of men and women, before decisions are taken (Beveridge *et al.* 2000a: 15). Central to this approach is the need to extend the participation of women within the policy-making process.

Gender mainstreaming came to widespread prominence when it featured in the Platform for Action of the Fourth World Conference on Women in Beijing in 1995. It emerged at the EU level in a number of areas. The Fourth Equal

Opportunities Action Programme (1996–2000) and 1996 Commission Communication *Incorporating Equal Opportunities for Women and Men into all Community Policies and Activities* committed the Commission to adopting a gender mainstreaming approach in respect of all Community policies (European Commission 1996). Gender mainstreaming was formally recognised in the 1997 Amsterdam Treaty, while the Commission has attempted to 'operationalise and consolidate' the gender mainstreaming approach through the adoption of a 2001–2005 framework strategy on gender equality.

In addition to this general commitment, the approach has also been aimed at specific policy areas. Article 1 of the new Framework Regulation for the Structural Funds (2000–2006) states that the EU should contribute to the 'elimination of inequalities and the promotion of equality between men and women' (Council of the European Union 1999b). Furthermore, Article 36 requires statistics for monitoring and evaluation purposes to be broken down by sex and Article 41 states that *ex ante* evaluation of national plans will include a gender impact assessment (Mazey 2001: 44). Meanwhile, the creation of the European Employment Strategy has also provided a window of opportunity to integrate mainstreaming approaches into the Community's policies. In 1999 a new Guideline was introduced under the Equal Opportunities Pillar requiring the member states 'to adopt a gender-mainstreaming approach in implementing the guidelines of all four pillars' (Council of the European Union 1999c).

Since 1997, Tony Blair's Labour Government has actively welcomed the gender mainstreaming method and developed a number of initiatives to promote its use in domestic governance. The Government claims that for women to become truly equal, they must become equally represented in key areas of public life (Women and Equality Unit (WEU) 2003: 14). At the 1997 general election, progress appeared to be made in this direction as the number of women MPs doubled from 60 to 120, partly due to the Labour Party's use of all-female shortlists during the selection process. Despite this increase, at just 18%, this proportion of women MPs is still among the lowest in Europe.

In light of the limited progress made in raising levels of female representation, increasing importance rests with the Government's efforts to directly incorporate a gender perspective into the policy-making process. Examples of this pledge to place women's issues 'firmly at the centre of government' include the creation of a Minister for Women and a Women's Unit. Their roles were to 'coordinate work across departments, so supporting ministers across Whitehall, in their efforts to promote women's interests' (Squires and Wickham-Jones 2002: 63). In November 1998, the Women's Unit issued new policy appraisal for equal treatment (PAET) guidelines to each Government department, designed to help policy makers consider the gender impact of any proposed policy (DWP 2002: 44).

Despite these changes it is clear the Labour Government has found the notion of mainstreaming difficult to incorporate in practice. During Labour's first term, the Women's Unit was seen as a weak and marginalised body with no real power base. Its mandate was deemed too broad and imprecise, its work was poorly aligned with the Government's broader political agenda, it enjoyed little publicity and it had little influence in directly shaping policy proposals (Squires and Wickham-Jones 2002: 63–8). Likewise the 1998 PAET guidelines have been heavily criticised for giving little genuine guidance to departments on how policy appraisals are to be conducted and for failing to establish machinery to monitor their effectiveness (Nott 1999: 215–17; Beveridge *et al.* 2000b: 186–8). Consequently, one expert concluded that the current PAET guidelines 'will not ensure that policy-making becomes transparent, accessible and responsive to women's situations' (Beveridge *et al.* 2000b: 189).

At present, even the Government admits that 'in many fields there is more to be done and there is still a long way to go' (WEU 2003: 11). To this end the DTI, working with the reformed Women and Equality Unit (WEU),[19] has recently announced a comprehensive strategy designed to bring about measurable improvements in gender equality across a range of indicators by 2006. For example, the strategy aims to achieve an overall balance of men and women on the boards of all public bodies by 2005. It also requires the WEU to work more closely with departments to encourage a gender impact analysis to be incorporated into their policy making (WEU 2003: 14–15). Interestingly, though central government has struggled to integrate gender mainstreaming techniques into the policy process, the devolved governments in Scotland, Wales and Northern Ireland appear to have performed far better in this respect. While all three regional assemblies have a formal statutory obligation to promote equality, they have all enthusiastically embraced the concept of mainstreaming and integrated and embedded it much more deeply into their policy-making processes (Beveridge *et al.* 2000c: 402–3; Mazey 2001: 53; Rees 2002: 14).

What remains less clear is the extent to which these changes, at both the national and regional levels, have been induced by the activities of the European Union. Generally, if the Government has given any acknowledgement to external bodies for the emergence of the gender mainstreaming technique, this has been to the United Nations rather than the EU (WEU 2003: 67). At the regional level, mainstreaming demands linked to EU structural funds have clearly played an important role. Overall, the UK has clearly been influenced by the emergence of a new indirect framework for conceptualising gender equality from external sources. This confirms that in accordance with the emergence of the previous two policy frameworks, the UK has generally followed rather than led advances in the way gender equality is conceptualised and pursued.

Conclusion

As the number of women entering the labour market has increased since the 1960s, so too have demands for workplace equality in order to overcome the numerous forms of direct and indirect discrimination that many women encountered. Though most changes occurred at the national level, political space emerged in the 1970s for the EU to champion some aspects of women's employment rights. By exploiting the existing Article 119 Treaty basis and promoting the development of a range of national and European-level institutional actors, the EU was able to develop a significant equal opportunities agenda. During three distinct waves of policy activism, the EU sought to improve the position of women within the labour market by advancing a range of hard laws and soft regulatory strategies. As a result, equal opportunity between men and women 'is one of the few policy areas where EU policy has outstripped the policy of the Member States' (Bagilhole 1997: 79). With one of the least developed gender policies, particularly in regard to workplace equal opportunities, the UK has been continually challenged by EU gender policy developments.

For the four Conservative Governments who served successive terms between 1979 and 1997, promoting 'equality of opportunity or even equal treatment' was not regarded as a strong 'social priority' (Bagilhole 1997: 95). Indeed, during these years the UK was able to prevent the adoption of much of the Commission's draft equal opportunities legislation, or at least its extension to Britain. Nevertheless, in the face of often intense ideological and practical opposition, the rulings of the ECJ have contributed to a major extension of the workplace rights, protections and entitlements accorded to British women. By establishing an explicit body of uniform European equality rights, Article 119 and the early gender Directives provided the Commission and private litigants with a solid legal basis to advance the principle of equal treatment within the Courts. Significantly, the ECJ generally interpreted these laws in an expansive and socially progressive manner.

Labour's decision to sign the Social Chapter on accession to office in May 1997 enabled the EU to extend the coverage of the directives on parental leave and part-time work to the UK, and adopt the Directive on fixed-term work. This decision signified the transition to a more consensual relationship between Britain and the EU. Tony Blair's Government proclaimed a far stronger commitment to the principle of equal opportunities than its Conservative pred-ecessor, especially in terms of developing a 'family-friendly' employment agenda. To implement these new gender Directives, Britain was again required to introduce a range of new statutory employment rights into areas previously outside of state regulation. However, the limited objectives and flexibility of the 'second wave' Directives provided the Government, and in some instances employers and employees themselves, with the scope to determine the level at which these new rights and entitlements would be set. Consequently, the Government introduced transposition regulations that, while broadly in accor-dance with the new European legal requirements, established a relatively low floor of minimum rights when compared with those enjoyed in other member states. Most recently, the EU's 'soft' regulatory approach to gender policy, exemplified by the equal opportunities 'pillar' in the European Employment Strategy and 'gender mainstreaming', has induced a degree of policy change in the UK, but only in areas where British and European agendas have coincided. However, as both the European Employment Strategy and gender mainstream-ing strategies intend to influence national policies over a longer time frame, immediate change should not be expected.

To conclude, the EU has had an uneven, but fundamental impact on British gender policy. While British women (and men) owe many of their recent statu-tory rights and entitlements to developments at the European level, the Conservative and Labour Governments' willingness to directly obstruct the adoption of European policies and limit the extent of domestic policy change has mitigated the potential impact of European agenda setting in gender policy. As seen elsewhere, this form of Europeanisation is very different from that found in other policy sectors.

Final point: why mainstreaming works for gender policy and not for others – a complexity perspective?

As discussed above, gender mainstreaming emerged at the EU level in the 1990s and became one of the most successful elements of EU gender policy. Using gender mainstreaming, gender policy promoters built upon the EU's fundamental treaty, legal structure and policy developments to push into completely new areas of policy. A very interesting point linked to this development was that gender actors were not the only ones to try and promote a mainstreaming strategy. Proponents of policies for disability and the elderly also attempted to use mainstreaming during this period, but much less successfully (Geyer 2000a). What was it that enabled gender actors to take advantage of this new strategy when others failed? From a complexity perspective there were several layered reasons.

At the most fundamental level, EU gender policy has a number of advantages over policies for disability and the elderly. It represents the interests of half the European population and voters, has experienced substantial intellectual and public recognition since the mid-20th century and has seen impressive policy growth in every member state. These advantages do not guarantee the success of gender policy initiatives, but greatly lower the barriers to them. At a less fundamental level, gender policy has a number of institutional advantages within the EU. It has a well-established treaty base, significant legal foundation in judicial decision making, notable history of QMV in the Council and access to a variety of EU level funding opportunities. Disability and elderly policy lack all of these advantages. Representing smaller groups with less wide-scale recognition, they have only recently been able to establish themselves within the core workings of the EU system.

Further, building on this fundamental strength, gender policy actors have been able to establish one of the largest social non-governmental organisations (NGOs) at the European level (the EWL) and maintain excellent linkages to the member state level through the activities of the EWL. The EWL has also been particularly active in legal/judicial areas, offering expertise and advice at both the EU and member state levels. Mainstreaming fits in well with the basic strategies of the EWL and their attempts to encourage and hold together the various member state-level women's organisations. At the same time, it gives them the opportunity to push gender issues into virtually any area of EU policy, radically expanding their potential sphere of activity. Finally, mainstreaming enhances the underlying narrative discourse of 'third wave' feminist thinking in that it goes beyond merely trying to make women equal to men in the sphere of labour policy, and opens up a whole range of issues and areas that can potentially challenge the gender relations underpinning the family, work–home life balance, the role of sex workers and much more (*see* Figure 6.1).

From this perspective it is easy to see that due to the fundamental advantages of gender policy within the EU system, gender policy actors were able to take advantage of the concepts of mainstreaming and successfully integrate it into its policy tactics. Other actors, lacking these fundamentals, were unable to fully take advantage of the mainstreaming strategy and integrate it into their policy tactics. In the long term, it does not guarantee gender policy. The fundamentals could alter, discourses may change and a backlash against the success of gender

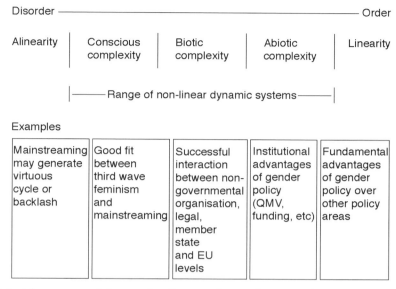

Figure 6.1 The range of dynamics for gender mainstreaming success.

mainstreaming could develop. However, given the reinforcing developments at each level of complexity for gender mainstreaming, it is likely that its success will continue.

Notes

1   Although Article 119 has since been amended and renumbered as Article 141, this chapter will refer to the original Treaty of Rome numbering throughout.
2   Council Directive 75/117/EEC.
3   Council Directive 76/207/EEC.
4   Council Directive 79/7/EEC.
5   Council Directive 86/378/EEC.
6   Council Directive 86/613/EEC.
7   (1982) ECR 2601.
8   *Hayward* v. *Cammell Laird* (1988) IRLR 257.
9   Article 119 was ruled to have *direct effect* in *Defrenne* v. *Sabena* (1976). The ETD was given *direct effect* in *Marshall* v. *Southampton and South-West Hampshire Area Health Authority (Teaching)* (1986).
10 Directive 96/34/EC on the framework agreement on parental leave concluded by UNICE, CEEP and the ETUC, 14 December 1995, was adopted unanimously on 3 June 1996 without debate in the Social Affairs Council.
11 Council Directive 97/81/EC. Extended to the UK by Council Directive 98/23/EC.
12 Council Directive 99/70/EC.
13 These changes were introduced by the Trade Union Reform and Employment Rights Act 1993. This amended the relevant provisions in the Employment Protection (Consolidation) Act 1978.
14 Recommendation 92/131/EEC of 27 November 1991.
15 Council Declaration 92/C27/01 of 19 December 1991.
16 Council Recommendation 92/241/EEC of 31 March 1992.

17 OJ 1986 C 176/79.

18 OJ 1997 C 394.

19 In June 2001 the Women's Unit was relaunched and renamed the Women and Equality Unit. It also moved from the Department of Social Security to the Cabinet Office.

Chapter 7

Regulating the labour market: the partial Europeanisation of British labour market policy

Since 1974, the European Commission's attempts to develop a more active European Union (EU) labour market policy have generated some of the greatest opposition to the process of European integration in Britain. In seeking to demonstrate that Europe had a 'social face' commensurate to its economic orientation at a time of growing social unrest, economic recession and industrial change, the 1974 Social Action Programme (SAP) proposed a series of European statutory rights to employee participation and employment protection. During the subsequent wave of EU policy activism in the mid-1970s and early 1980s, the Commission sought to develop a harmonised body of European labour law based on the highly regulated Romano-Germanic system of industrial relations. Yet while a strategy of upward harmonisation posed few problems for the numerically dominant members of the 'continental' model, it presented a far greater challenge to Britain's voluntaristic industrial relations tradition where outside of core areas like workplace health and safety, British workers have traditionally had little statutory protection, or 'labour law,' to safeguard their rights. The divisions between these two traditions and the Rome Treaty requirement of unanimous voting on all labour market directives meant that only three narrow Directives were adopted during this period.

By contrast, during a 'second wave' of European policy activism beginning in the early 1990s, the Commission managed to secure the adoption of many of its long-standing policy objectives. This followed a series of influential Treaty revisions that removed Britain's veto rights from a number of policy areas, but also reflected a major change in policy approach from both the Commission and the new Labour Government. First, the Commission came to accept that in a diversifying and expanding Community, the upward harmonisation of labour and social standards was increasingly inappropriate and instead sought the introduction of minimum standards. Hence, new EU labour legislation contained more limited objectives and provided far greater scope for the member states to implement the directives in accordance with existing national practices and traditions. Second, in stark contrast to the previous Conservative administration, Labour viewed the Social Chapter not as a pernicious 'European jobs tax' (John Major in Gowland and Turner 2000: 288), but 'as a sensible procedure for setting certain Europe-wide minimum standards' (The Labour Party 1997b). In this way, the objectives contained within the Social Chapter meshed well with Labour's broader third way agenda, part of which sought to reform core aspects of Britain's system of industrial relations. Together, these developments enabled the adoption of important Directives relating to the organisation of working time and the right for workers to be informed and consulted on a range of workplace issues.

Overall, the adoption of EU labour law directives has had an important twofold effect on Britain's labour market policy and system of industrial relations. They have contributed to a major extension of statutory regulation in British industrial relations and helped to establish minimum, though relatively low, levels of legal rights, protections and entitlements. However, the influence of EU labour law remains narrow. Moreover, many recent developments in British labour market policy are attributable to a nationally constructed reform agenda, rather than as a result of any formal adaptational pressure exerted by EU labour law.

The British voluntarist tradition of industrial relations

Fundamentally, Britain's opposition to and reluctant implementation of European labour law was attributable to the distinctiveness of the UK's 'voluntarist' industrial relations tradition. During the early period of rapid industrialisation, the employment relationship in Britain generally came to be governed by informal agreements between managers and workers at workplace level. With the emerging trade unions keen to avoid any 'hostile intervention of the courts in industrial disputes' and employers wishing to avoid any legislation that would constrain their 'freedom to manage', the absence of legal regulation in industrial relations was supported by both sides of industry (Edwards *et al.* 1992: 2–6). The adoption of the influential Trades Disputes Act in 1906 secured the right for trade unions to organise, bargain and take industrial action by establishing a series of *negative* immunities from common law liabilities. This helped ensure the primacy of voluntary collective bargaining in determining the rules of employment whereby, 'the policy of the state was not to regulate the terms and conditions of those who could protect themselves by collective action' (Hepple 1998: 238), and where collective agreements were not legally binding within the courts and were seen as no more than a 'gentleman's agreement' (Edwards 1995: 6–7). Moreover trade union recognition by employers was voluntary and the state provided little in the way of dispute resolution facilities (Goodman *et al.* 1998: 42–3).

As is well known, by the mid-1960s mounting industrial relations difficulties were increasingly undermining economic performance. As Britain continued its relative economic decline, many commentators apportioned blame for these difficulties on the voluntarist tradition. For the left, the system needed greater state involvement and workers' rights and should be modelled on the more organised and corporatist continental system. For the right, the problem was the power, restrictive practices and unofficial industrial action of the trade unions. Edward Heath's Conservative Government responded by introducing the 1971 Industrial Relations Act. This far-reaching legislation sought to reform bargaining structures, secure recognition of unions by employers and encourage legally enforceable collective agreements. Although these elements of the Act proved unacceptable to the unions and were later repealed by the newly elected Labour Government in 1974, the state became increasingly active in other areas of industrial relations. As part of the Labour Government's corporatist 'social contract' with the Trades Union Congress (TUC), the trade unions agreed to restraint in pay bargaining in return for a range of new legal rights for trade unions and workers (Hepple 1998). These included new legislation to improve health and safety at work and protections against unfair dismissal. During this period the Advisory Conciliation and Arbitration Service (ACAS) and Central Arbitration Committee (CAC) were also established, and the system of wages councils was strengthened.

The election of Margaret Thatcher's Conservative Government in 1979 marked a decisive shift in state intervention in labour markets. The principal aim of the Conservatives' reforms was 'to bolster employers' "right to manage" and promote greater flexibility in the labour market', to improve UK competitiveness and encourage employment growth (Milward *et al.* 1998: 10–11). This was achieved by a progressive weakening of statutory employment protections and a 'gradual tightening of restrictions on the activities of trade unions' (Milward *et al.* 1998: 10–11). These changes, introduced through seven Acts of Parliament adopted between 1980 and 1993, progressively restricted unions' rights to enforce closed shops and take secondary action, introduced new rules for the function, timing and nature of industrial ballots, weakened individuals' rights in relation to unfair dismissal and restricted the scope of the wages council (Hanson 1991; Goodman *et al.* 1998: 61–2).

The result of these various changes spelled the end of attempts to make the British system more corporatistic, reasserted the central role of the state in British labour relations and saw that the law 'became far more prevalent in British industrial relations' due to a series of nationally induced legislative changes introduced by both Labour and Conservative Governments (Edwards *et al.* 1992: 17). By the latter 1990s, the only truly 'voluntarist' aspect of the industrial relations system concerned the conduct or outcome of collective bargaining (Farnham and Pimlott 1995: 212–17). However, despite this complex pattern of change, Britain's system of industrial relations and labour market policy continued to exhibit a number of distinctive characteristics compared to the dominant traditions of its major European partners. These differences were central to the UK's inability to adapt to the 'first wave' labour law Directives.

The 'first wave' of European employee participation legislation

For Britain, the most controversial proposals to emanate from the 1974 SAP concerned the statutory regulation of employee participation. Employee participation is a term that embodies a range of ideas and concepts concerning how workers are integrated into the decision-making procedures of the company in which they work – it may also be termed industrial democracy (Gladstone 1993). Statutory rights for employee participation feature prominently in the more corporatist Romano-Germanic model of industrial relations. German workers, in particular, enjoy the strongest rights in Europe through the country's powerful co-determination laws (Marginson and Sisson 1994: 31–2). By contrast, the UK has no such tradition of statutory employee participation. In accordance with Britain's 'voluntarist' industrial relations system, workplace information and consultation was traditionally seen as a private matter between employer and employee. Consequently, the British Government and business community vehemently opposed a succession of European proposals for statutory employee participation during the 1970s and 1980s.

In 1975 the Commission published the draft European Company Statute (ECS). The proposal sought to give companies the option of forming a European Company (or Societas Europaea, SE) governed by European rather than national law (European Industrial Relations Observatory (EIRO) 2002d). The intention was to create a harmonised European legal framework to facilitate cross-border mergers and transnational cooperation between firms. As an economic proposal it was uncontroversial. However, its labour policy implications were significant and divisive (Tsoukalis 1993: 168). In particular, those countries with the strongest attachment to industrial democracy feared that if the European proposals undercut their existing national provisions, then domestic firms would be able to bypass these more stringent requirements by establishing themselves under European law (Rehfeldt, in Müller and Hoffmann 2001: 14). As a result, the Commission advocated the harmonisation of employee participation procedures to those standards enjoyed under the strongest national legislation and applied to all public limited companies with over 500 employees. These proposals, the early European Company Statute (ECS) Directive and 1972 'fifth' company law Directive, required the relevant companies to include employee representatives on supervisory boards with employees acting as full board members on a range of issues, and owed much to German conceptions of industrial democracy. In 1980 the Commission also published the draft 'Vredeling' Directive that sought to provide enhanced information and consultation rights to employees in multinational companies with over 100 workers (Cressey 1993; Geyer and Springer 1998).

As these measures were based on Article 100 of the Rome Treaty, requiring unanimous approval within the Council, all were obstructed by the British veto. This opposition forced the Commission to launch an arduous process of revision and amendment as the more ambitious elements of the proposed legislation were jettisoned. New drafts of the ECS were published in 1975, 1989 and 1991, while further drafts of the 'fifth' and Vredeling Directives were issued in 1983. However, in 1979 the newly elected Government of Margaret Thatcher remained immovable on the matter. Seeing compulsory employee participation as a gross infringement on managerial prerogative, the Conservatives firmly rejected what they deemed 'the imposition of failed policies of the 1970s' and 'socialism by the backdoor' (Cressey 1993: 86).

Although these attempts to introduce a general harmonised framework for employee participation within European corporate decision-making structures proved unsuccessful, the period did witness the adoption of three narrower Directives that sought to increase the legal protections afforded to workers in the context of major corporate restructuring across Europe. Under two of them, the new rights to employment protection were to be attained primarily through the introduction of minimum requirements for companies to inform and consult workers' representatives under a number of specific circumstances (Hall 1992: 1). During this period, therefore, legislative progress was achieved on the basis of the 'lowest common denominator' in Council of Minister negotiations (Hall 1994: 283).

The first European 'labour law' Directive to be adopted was the 1975 Collective Redundancies Directive (CRD).[1] This was followed in 1977 by a Directive designed to safeguard the rights of employees in the event of transfers of undertakings; also known as the Acquired Rights Directive (ARD).[2] Both Directives were motivated by heightened concerns of social dumping in the context of a rapidly changing European market, and required companies to inform and consult employees' representatives to help mitigate the potentially harmful consequences of planned redundancies or changing ownership structures.

Although the original CRD was marginally strengthened by amendments introduced in 1992, its requirements are relatively limited. Article 1 offers member states a range of options for defining a collective redundancy. Thereafter, the Directive requires those employers who are contemplating collective redundancies to supply the worker's representatives with all relevant information concerning those redundancies (Article 2.3). The subsequent consultation must be undertaken 'with a view to reaching an agreement' (Article 2.1), and should at least cover ways of avoiding the redundancies or reducing the number of workers affected (Article 2.2). Employers are also required to notify the 'competent public authority' of any projected redundancies (Article 3.1); these must not take effect earlier than 30 days after notification has been given (Article 4.1). Significantly, the Directive makes no reference of measures for enforcing these rights. For these reasons the CRD can mainly be seen as establishing a set of procedural rights for managing collective redundancies, rather than developing a substantive body of individual employment protection rights (Szyszczak 2000a: 112).

The information and consultation requirements contained under Article 6 of the ARD are similar to those of the CRD. Again, information must be provided in good time before the transfer is carried out and with a view to seeking agreement. However, unlike the CRD it also provides specific individual rights and obligations. Based upon French law, the ARD aims to protect the workers from dismissal as a result of the transfer of a business (Article 4), and allow employees to continue working under the same terms and conditions for the new employer (Article 3) (Szyszczak 2000b). Although the rights contained in the 1977 Directive, later modified in 1998,[3] were far weaker than those contained in the Commission's earlier proposals, EU case law has made the directive one of the most controversial pieces of EU labour law.

Finally, adopted in 1980, the Insolvency Directive was the third labour law Directive to successfully emerge from the 1974 Social Action Programme.[4] Based on the notion that the functioning of the common market may lead to increased bankruptcies and insolvencies, the Directive tried to provide protection for employees in the event of the insolvency of their employer (Blanpain and Engels 1998: 354). In particular it aimed to guarantee employees payment of their outstanding claims resulting from a contract of employment or employment relationship, relating to pay for the period prior to a given date specified by the member states (Szyszczak 2000a).

Implementing the directives: a clash of industrial cultures

Of the three directives, the adoption and implementation of the Insolvency Directive was uncomplicated and aroused comparatively little interest in the UK. Indeed, the Directive was generally welcomed in Britain, as its provisions were largely similar to existing UK legal requirements (Burrows and Mair 1996: 236).[5] However, complying with the terms of the directives on collective redundancies and acquired rights was far more problematic.

By introducing provisions that ran contrary to the 'established principles of the law of contract', incorporating the provisions of the ARD into UK law was a huge challenge for Britain (Burrows and Mair 1996: 177). The Conservative Government reluctantly implemented the ARD, after the transposition deadline, through the Transfer of Undertakings (Protection of Employment) Regulations 1981 (The 'TUPE' Regulations). A leading labour policy expert claimed that the TUPE Regulations represented 'perhaps the clearest example of the UK Government's minimalist approach to [implementing] EC labour law' (Bercusson 1996: 30). Following a 1992 Commission Implementation Report that highlighted a number of weaknesses in the TUPE Regulations, the Commission initiated legal proceedings against the British within the European Court of Justice (ECJ) on the basis of Article 169 of the Rome Treaty. Similarly, although the requirements of the CRD were relatively modest and many of its provisions were already catered for in UK employment law, the Commission again felt compelled to commence infringement proceedings against the UK for inadequate implementation of the CRD.[6]

Likewise the Commission's criticisms of the British legislation were also remarkably similar. The first complaint centred on the basic definitions given within the British legislation. For example, by excluding 'non-commercial ventures' from the scope of the TUPE Regulations, the Commission claimed this severely narrowed the protections afforded to British workers and contravened the terms of the ARD. In particular it enabled private contractors to compete for the provision of former public services by reducing the pay and standards of existing workers following a transfer. Given that public services were defined as non-commercial ventures by the original Regulations, this exclusion was particularly damaging for a large number of public sector workers in the context of the Conservative's privatisation policy during the 1980s (Bercusson 1996). Similarly, the Commission was critical of the narrow definition of redundancy given within the 1992 (Consolidation) Act intended to give legal effect to the CRD. The Conservative Government responded by broadening the definition of redundancy in 1993.

Another example identified by the Commission concerned the nature of the consultation to be undertaken. Under both the CRD and ARD, employers' consultations with the workers' representatives must be undertaken 'with a view to reaching an agreement'.[7] The Commission argued that the British legislation failed to adequately incorporate this, thereby significantly weakening the potential benefits that could be derived from informing and consulting with workers' representatives. Both the TUPE Regulations and the 1992 (Consolidation) Act have since been amended to comply with this requirement. For example, following an employer's announcement of collective redundancies, the Regulations now require consultation that actively seeks ways to avoid the dismissals or reduce the number of employees to be dismissed, and endeavours to mitigate the effects of these dismissals (Burrows and Mair 1996: 218–19).

Although the British Government had amended its transposition legislation in response to the majority of the Commission's criticisms *before* the ECJ had delivered its rulings, one criticism remained unresolved at the time of the Court's judgements. Both directives required the giving of information to and consultation of *workers' representatives* in the event of collective redundancies or the transfer of an undertaking. However, at the time the UK had no tradition of institutionalised workforce consultation that was common in other systems (EIRO 1999d). Indeed, the UK and Ireland were the only member states 'without a generally-applicable system of information and consultation through works councils or similar bodies established by law or collective agreement' (EIRO 1997b: 2). Although at the time of the Directives' adoption the UK *did* have in place legal procedures that could require employers to recognise their workers' representatives,[8] the 1979 Conservative Government repealed these procedures in line with its policy of de-collectivisation in British industrial relations (Bercusson 1996: 30). The Commission therefore argued that in the absence of voluntary trade union recognition by an employer for purposes of collective bargaining, the British legislation provided no means for the selection of non-union employee representation for consultative purposes in line with the directives' requirements and rendered the directives provisions largely ineffective for a considerable proportion of the British workforce, especially given the declining extent of trade union recognition and union-based bargaining (Hepple 1998: 240). This deficiency was confirmed by the influential Workplace Industrial Relations Survey that charted the emergence of a significant 'representation gap' (Hall in EIRO 1997b; Terry in EIRO 1999d) in British industrial relations.

In two judgements, the ECJ in *European Commission* v. *UK* (1994)[9] ruled that the British legislation breached the terms of the CRD and ARD. Although the Court stressed the UK was not required to introduce compulsory trade union recognition, it did require the UK to introduce procedures for the selection of non-union representation for consultation purposes in accordance with the terms of the directives. The Conservative Government reluctantly responded in 1995 by introducing new regulations that required employers to consult with representatives of recognised unions *or* other representatives elected by the workforce, in the event of impending redundancies or transfers. However, if a workplace had both trade union representatives *and* elected representatives, the employer was permitted to consult with either, thereby threatening to undermine recognised independent trade unions (Hepple 1998: 240). Furthermore, the 1995 Amendment Regulations made no provision for permanent worker representatives, nor were the procedures for the election of these representatives established (European Industrial Relations Review (EIRR) 1996).

Unsurprisingly, the 1995 Regulations were strongly criticised by the trade unions, while the Commission complained that the regulations still did not fully conform to the Court's ruling. The 1997 Blair Government supported these arguments and introduced further amendments in 1999 designed to make the legislation 'clearer and easier to understand and comply with' (Department of Trade and Industry (DTI) 1999a). Under the 1999 Regulations a number of significant changes have been introduced. Firstly, if employees who may be affected are represented by an independent trade union recognised for purposes of collective bargaining, the employer is no longer permitted to bypass this union in favour of consultation with other employee representatives. This change gives an important boost to existing forms of union representation. Secondly, the Regulations establish clear and explicit rules for the election of employee representatives in non-union firms. Thirdly, the amount of compensation to be paid by the employer in the event of non-compliance has been increased. If an employer has failed to properly inform or consult with its workforce, a tribunal can now award 90 days' pay in all cases involving collective redundancies, and 13 weeks' pay in cases involving transfers of undertakings.

Overall, that Britain was still amending its implementing legislation nearly a quarter of a century after the adoption of the original Directives demonstrates that Britain has been very reluctant to undertake the considerable domestic policy adaptation needed in order to comply with European law in these areas, and illustrates the difficulty of separating UK and EU dynamics. On the one hand, the actions of the Commission and ECJ eventually forced Britain to amend its statute law to create an *ad hoc* system for consulting employees' representatives in the absence of recognised trade unions (Goodman *et al.* 1998: 59). On the other hand, the delaying tactics of the Conservatives led to 'long periods during which EC labour law has failed to operate as it should in the UK' (Bercusson 1996: 31). Under Labour there is now greater clarity between the terms of the Directives and the British Regulations as the party portrays itself as a stronger supporter of these consultation rights than its Conservative predecessor. Nevertheless, following a number of high-profile cases of company restructuring (the 2000 break-up and sale of the Rover Group by BMW and the closure of the Vauxhall Plant in Luton by GM), the Labour Government announced its intention to, once again, review the UK's employee consultation requirements relating to collective redundancies, demonstrating that the process of UK–EU industrial relations adaptation is far from over.

The 'second wave': working time and employee participation

Following the publication of the 1989 Social Charter and action programme, and the Treaty's revision at Maastricht, a second generation of EU labour law emerged. In addition to directives on part-time and fixed-term working and amendments made to the Directives on acquired rights and collective redundancies, the 1990s saw the adoption of directives on the proof of employment,[10] the rights of 'posted' workers,[11] and the protection of young workers.[12] The most significant of this 'second wave' of directives concerned the regulation of working time and employee participation. In both policy areas the UK had little or no prior experience of statutory regulation. Although the adoption of these directives represented a radical departure for UK employment law, the 1993 Working Time Directive (WTD), 1994 European Works Councils Directive (EWCD) and 2002 national-level Information and Consultation Directive (ICD) were all concerned with establishing minimum requirements and were far narrower than earlier Commission proposals. Furthermore, these Directives provided considerable scope for the member states to derogate from a number of core requirements and delegate the task of elaborating the detailed provisions to management and labour (Bercusson 1996: 306).

The Working Time Directive

Contrary to the statutory working time legislation prevalent in most European states, working time arrangements in Britain have traditionally been determined in a voluntaristic manner through bargaining between management and labour and governed by individual contracts of employment. Following the ruling in *Tucker* v. *British Leyland Motor Co. Ltd* (1978), English common law provided no restrictions on the number of hours that could be worked or any entitlements to holiday (Adnett and Hardy 2001: 121). Furthermore, as part of its programme of labour market deregulation, the Conservative Government during the 1980s presided over the abolition of the few existing statutory rules governing specific issues of working time (Burrows and Mair 1996: 282).[13] Consequently, when the Commission revived proposals for the Europe-wide regulation of working time in the Social Charter, the UK Government remained fiercely opposed. This opposition was compounded by evidence of significant structural differences between British and continental working patterns. The Government feared that together these factors could make compliance with any European regulation both difficult and costly. Studies revealed that full-time workers in Britain work the highest number of hours in the EU, between 3 and 5 hours more per week than their EU counterparts. The British also had the highest percentage (around 16%) of workers working over 48 hours a week and the most employed on shift and night work (Burrows and Mair 1996).

Recognising the resolute opposition of the UK, the Commission chose to present and defend working time regulation in terms of protecting the health and safety of workers that could be determined in the Council under qualified majority voting (QMV) procedures. As such, the preamble to the (draft) Working Time Directive referred to the possible detrimental effects to health posed by shift working, night working and the working of excessively long hours, and the legal basis of the draft proposal was Article 118a (health and safety).[14] This 'Trojan horse' strategy (Geyer 2000a) enabled the Commission to obtain QMV status for the WTD, surmount the UK opposition and pass the Directive in November 1993.

In response, the British Government initiated legal proceedings against the Council to challenge the legality of the Directive's Treaty base in health and safety, arguing instead that it should have been based on Article 100a, which specifically refers to the 'rights and interests of employed persons' and is subject to a unanimous vote. The Government demanded that the ECJ annul the main substantive provisions of the WTD and refused to begin transposition until the ECJ had delivered its verdict. However, the Court rejected the British case, ruling that:

> There is nothing in the wording of Article 118a to indicate that the concepts of 'working environment', 'safety' and 'health' as used in that provision should ... be interpreted restrictively, and not as embracing all factors, phys-

ical or otherwise, capable of affecting the health and safety of the worker in his working environment, including in particular certain aspects of the organisation of working time (Case C-84/94 *UK* v. *Council* (1996) ECR I-5755).

Following this judgement the British Government was legally obliged to give effect to the provisions of the WTD within UK law.

In using Article 118a as the legal basis for the WTD, the Commission had successfully surmounted UK opposition, but was limited to the adoption of minimum requirements, thereby ensuring that the Treaty basis could not be used as a 'vehicle for upward harmonisation' (Moffat 1998: 16). As a result, the 1993 Working Time Directive provided for minimum *entitlements* to:

- **daily rest:** minimum daily rest period of 11 consecutive hours per 24-hour period (Article 3) and a rest break during a 6-hour working day (Article 4)
- **weekly rest:** an uninterrupted 24-hour rest period every week (Article 5)
- **annual leave:** 4 weeks' annual paid leave (Article 7)
- **average weekly working time:** average weekly working time, including overtime, should not exceed 48 hours (Article 6)
- **night work:** is not permitted to exceed an average of 8 hours in any 24-hour period (Article 8). Night workers are also entitled to free and regular health assessments, and where possible must be transferred to day shifts where health problems connected with night shift working arise (Article 9).

However, having established this body of minimum limits and entitlements, the Directive proceeded to list an extensive range of member state derogations that some commentators argued rendered many of the provisions 'of doubtful value'. These provisions included:

- **general exclusions:** under Article 1.1(3) workers in air, rail, road, sea, inland waterway and lake transport, sea fishing, other work at sea and the activities of doctors in training were excluded from the Directive[15]
- **reference periods:** under Article 16, member states were accorded considerable discretion in setting reference periods for calculating average working times for the application of Articles 5 (weekly rest), 6 (maximum weekly working time), and 8 (night work)
- **derogations:** Article 17 permitted member states to derogate from the minimum legal standards set by the Directive in three main instances:
  - where the duration of working time is not measured and/or can be predetermined by the workers themselves (e.g. managing executives)
  - in occupations, work activities or situations which are expressly provided for by the Directive
  - where a workforce or collective agreement(s) has been reached to amplify or restrict the coverage of particular provisions in relation to working time (Adnett and Hardy 2001: 121).
- **voluntary exemption:** Article 18, included at the behest of the UK Government, permitted member states to 'opt-out' from the 48-hour limit on the average working week contained under Article 6 if the workers concerned agreed to the exemption and the employers kept detailed records

of the working practices. Given the number of workers in the UK working in excess of 48 hours per week, there were significant concerns over the negative implications this limit could have on British working practices (Moffat 1998: 24).

The European Works Councils and Information and Consultation Directives

As seen earlier, the absence of any prior statutory procedures for informing and consulting workers in the UK made compliance with the Directives on 'acquired rights' and collective redundancies particularly problematic and also helps account for the British Government's hostility towards the more substantive Romano-Germanic-inspired employee participation proposals of the 1970s. Yet while the draft ECS, 'fifth' and Vredeling Directives had all successfully been obstructed by the British veto in the 1980s, by the early 1990s developments arising from the single market programme had created a window of opportunity for the Commission to revive proposals for statutory employee participation.

In the context of the growing transnationalisation of corporate structures, the Commission argued that nationally defined rights to information and consultation, enjoyed by employees in all member states apart from the UK and Ireland, were becoming increasingly ineffectual when decisions were being taken in a different country to that of its workers (Hall 1992: 2–3). Furthermore, given that significant corporate restructuring often follows in the wake of mergers or take-overs, it was felt this was a time when employees were most in need of rights to participate in decisions affecting their futures. Hoover's infamous decision to relocate from Spain to Scotland in 1993 served only to exacerbate fears of 'social dumping' by large multinational companies (Geyer and Springer 1998). Therefore, with companies increasingly operating on a transnational footing, the Commission argued they also needed to be regulated at a transnational level (Marginson and Sisson 1994: 15).

In contrast to the more ambitious proposals issued during the 'first wave', the draft EWCD was concerned solely with establishing a floor of minimum rights in relation to *transnational* information and consultation arrangements, thereby ensuring that national-level traditions and practices could be maintained. Indeed Wolfgang Streeck argued that European Works Councils (EWCs) are best understood, not as the creation of general European institutions, 'but as the international extension of national industrial relations systems that continue to remain distinctly different' (Streeck 1998: 446). Over time, it was hoped this approach would help the EU develop a distinct identity in the sphere of transnational employee participation (Hall 1994: 293).

Despite these modifications, the British Conservative Government retained its intransigent stance arguing that the proposals constituted a 'breach of voluntarism', were 'alien to the UK tradition' and would affect UK firms much more than European ones. Given this continued opposition, the Commission exploited the new Social Protocol procedures agreed at Maastricht (requiring only QMV in the Council) to bypass the British veto, and successfully passed the EWC directive (Directive 94/45/EEC). Having been adopted under the terms of the Social Protocol, Britain was not required to transpose the EWCD into British law, although a significant number of British-owned companies were required to comply with the Directive by virtue of exceeding the employee thresholds in two or more participating states. Later circumstances dictated that this anomalous position was to prove relatively short-lived, as the Labour Government signed the Social Chapter on accession to office in 1997. Consequently, the EWCD was extended to Britain by way of a separate Directive signed on 15 December 1997. As with the original Directive, a two-year period was provided for the UK to adopt the necessary transposition legislation.

Following its adoption, former Social Affairs Commissioner Padraig Flynn hailed the EWCD as 'a Directive of the new generation; a real framework Directive'. He argued that it characterised the increasingly flexible nature of EU labour law by allowing member states to preserve national industrial relations practices and permitting companies to find 'tailored solutions which suit their situations best' (in Colaianni 1996: ix). However, other commentators focused on the EWCD's relatively limited rights to information and consultation, and argued that unless management and labour voluntarily negotiate worthwhile agreements then the EWCD would only be of symbolic value (Müller and Hoffmann 2001: 36).

The basic elements of the EWCD included:

- **objective:** to improve the rights to information and consultation of employees in Community-scale undertakings and groups of undertakings. This requires the establishment of a European Works Council or appropriate alternative procedure for informing and consulting workers in every Community-scale undertaking or groups of undertakings (Article 2.1(f))
- **enterprises affected:** all 'Community-scale' undertakings and groups of undertakings with at least 1000 employees across the member states including at least 150 workers employed in each of two or more member states (Article 2).[16] The TUC estimated that during the British opt-out, 116 were covered by the scope of the 1994 EWCD. Following the adoption of the 1997 Extension Directive a further 111 British firms were included (TUC 1998: 94)
- **existing voluntary agreements:** arrangements tailored to the circumstances of the enterprise are prioritised (Carley and Hall 2000: 105). As such, Article 13 states that companies are exempt if there is an agreement in place 'covering the entire workforce, providing for the transnational information and consultation or employees'
- **negotiation procedure:** if no 'Article 13' agreement exists, Article 5 rules that the process of establishing an EWC, or alternative information and consultation procedure, can be initiated either by central management or at the request of at least 100 employees from more than one country. A 'special negotiating body' (SNB) of employee representatives will be established to negotiate a written agreement with central management and determine the 'scope, composition, functions and term of office of the European Works Council' or alternative information and consultation procedure (Hall *et al.* 1995: 6)
- **subsidiary requirements:** contained in the Annex to the Directive, determine that an EWC is to be established on the basis of a number of standard rules that govern an EWC's competence, composition, information and consultation rights and operating expenses.

In recent years, the EU has successfully extended its statutory information and consultation rights through the adoption of two further Council Directives. Firstly, in October 2001 the Council of Ministers adopted a Regulation to establish a European Company Statute (ECS) and an accompanying Directive concerning employee participation in the new European Companies (Societas Europaea, SE).[17] Should a company operating in more than one member state voluntarily establish itself as a new European company based in European rather than national law, the Directive provides for European-level information and consultation arrangements in the new SE. Where no agreement is reached between management and employee representatives a set of statutory 'standard rules' is applied, in certain circumstances this includes board-level employee participation (EIRO 2002d). As seen earlier the first such proposal was made almost 30 years ago.

Secondly, and of greater significance for British labour market policy, in March 2002 the Council adopted Information and Consultation Directive 2002/14/EC 'establishing a general framework for informing and consulting employees'. The Commission first submitted a draft Directive to extend information and consultation rights to the national level in November 1998 following the controversial closure of the Renault plant in Vilvoorde, Belgium, with the loss of 3160 jobs (European Works Councils Bulletin (EWCB) 1997: 10). This, the Commission argued, highlighted that the existing laws on employee participation at the national and Community levels were both fragmented and ineffectual. Moreover, the Commission also claimed that reinforcing mechanisms for employee participation could serve a productive role in assisting the modernisation of work organisation (Barnard 2000a: 540).

In Britain the proposal generated deep divisions between the employers' organisations and the trade unions (EIRO 2002c). Whereas the TUC was strongly in favour, the Confederation of British Industry (CBI) branded the draft Directive as a 'completely unacceptable breach of the principle of subsidiarity' (EIRO 1999b). Indeed the CBI's opposition was largely responsible for the Union des Industries de la Communauté Européene's (UNICE's) resistance towards negotiating a Social Partner agreement, despite the support of the European Trade Union Confederation (ETUC) and CEEP. Although the new Labour Government was a firmer supporter of EU labour market policy in general, the 1998 *Fairness At Work* White Paper also claimed it was difficult to reconcile the proposal with the principle of subsidiarity and that the Directive 'would cut across existing practices in member states to no benefit' (DTI 1998: 4.5). However, following the controversial break-up of the Rover Group and the announcement of significant job losses in the wake of the closure of Vauxhall's Luton plant, pressure mounted on the Government to drop its opposition to the national information and consultation Directive. During the negotiations that ensued, the Government managed to secure a number of important amendments to the original draft proposal. Consequently, although the CBI was 'deeply disappointed by the agreement of this dossier', it has praised the Government for negotiating the least damaging option (CBI 2001a; CBI 2001b).

The IC Directive applies to all undertakings with at least 50 employees in any one member state or, at the choice of individual national governments, establishments with at least 20 employees (Article 3.1). These undertakings or establishments must inform and consult employee representatives about the recent and probable development of their activities and economic situation, the possible threat to employment, and any substantial changes in work organisation or in contractual relations (Article 4.2). As with the EWCD, the 2002 Directive establishes some basic requirements for the nature, method and timing of information and consultation (Article 4.3, 4.4), but states that the practical arrangements are to be defined and implemented in accordance with national law and industrial relations practice in individual member states (Article 1.2). Likewise, the Directive allows management and labour at the undertaking or establishment level to conclude agreements to determine the practical arrangements for informing and consulting employees. These agreements, and pre-existing agreements concluded before the Directive's transposition deadline, may establish provisions that are different from those referred to in Article 4 (Article 5). While the Directive must be transposed into national legislation by 23 March 2005, Article 10 enables member states without established statutory systems of employee information and consultation (effectively the UK and Ireland) to phase in the coverage of the Directive (EIRO 2002a).[18]

Implementing the 'second wave'

Following victory at the 1997 general election the incoming Labour Government was legally obliged to implement the 1994 WTD. However, by honouring its manifesto pledge to sign the Social Chapter, the Government was also required to give legal effect to the EWCD. As these Directives have required the introduction of statutory employment rights into the previously unregulated areas of working time and employee participation, these 'second wave' European labour market Directives have had a significant effect on two core areas of British industrial relations. Yet although the Directives have exposed British policy to strong forces of vertical Europeanisation and contributed to a significant extension of statutory regulation in British industrial relations, Labour's transposition legislation is notable for having established a relatively low level of legal rights, protections and entitlements. On the one hand this is attributable to the relatively limited objectives of the 'second wave' labour law Directives. On the other hand it reflects the fact that the Labour Government has made generous use of the derogations and exceptions provided by the Directives, in an attempt to strike a delicate balance between further extending UK employment rights and maintaining flexibility and competitiveness.

Implementing the Working Time Directive

The Working Time Regulations (WTR), introduced to implement the Community's WTD, came into effect on 1 October 1998 – nearly two years after the Directives' transposition deadline.[19] This delay was largely attributable to the Conservatives' ultimately unsuccessful challenge to the legal basis of the WTD and the change of government in 1997. In close accordance with the minimum provisions of the Directive, the WTR provide a number of basic rights and protections including a 48-hour working week, entitlement to four weeks' annual paid holiday, rights to rest breaks and rest periods, limits to night work and free health assessments for night workers.

To the dismay of the UK trade unions, in formulating the WTR the new Labour Government took full advantage of the derogations and exemptions in the WTD – a fact largely welcomed by the CBI (Lourie 1998: 23; Goss and Adam-Smith 2001: 197). Most significantly, Britain was the only member state to make use of the Directive's provision for an individual opt-out from the statutory limit on weekly working time. This differs markedly from the French Government's initial implementation of the WTD in which they far exceeded the minimum requirements of the WTD by reducing the standard French 'working week' from 39 to 35 hours (Adnett and Hardy 2001: 120). The UK Regulations also fully exploit the opportunities provided by Article 17 to derogate from the Directive's provisions on rest breaks, daily and weekly rest periods, night work and reference periods.

Since the Regulations were adopted in 1998, the Labour Government has introduced a number of changes to its original transposition legislation. Although the Government effectively pursued a minimalist approach towards implementing the WTD, claims from the British business community that certain provisions had been enhanced or 'gold-plated' prompted the introduction of amendment Regulations in 1999 (Barnard 2000b: 167). When first issued, the Regulations were widely regarded 'as one of the most complex pieces of employment legislation ever faced by UK employers' (EIRO 1998). In particular, the main criticism concerned the extensive and bureaucratic record-keeping requirements placed on employers in relation to those workers who had signed an 'individual opt-out' from the 48-hour average weekly working limit. The 1999 amendment Regulations have since replaced the earlier detailed record-keeping requirements with a simple obligation to keep an up-to-date list of those workers who have signed an opt-out (EIRO 1999f).

However, following a successful legal challenge to the adequacy of Britain's implementing legislation, the Labour Government has also been formally required to strengthen certain aspects of the UK Regulations. In January 1999, the British High Court made an Article 177 referral to the ECJ following a challenge to the adequacy of the holiday entitlement provisions established under the Regulations (EIRO 2001d). By entitling workers to annual paid leave only after 13 weeks' continuous employment with the same employer, the Broadcasting, Entertainment, Cinematograph and Theatre Union (BECTU) claimed the WTR breached the automatic entitlement to annual paid leave contained within the Directive. The ECJ upheld the trade union's complaint in June 2001 by noting that the Directive provides no scope for derogating from the 'unconditional' annual leave entitlement contained under Article 7.1 (EIRO, July 2001c).[20] Consequently, the WTR were amended in October 2001 to give workers in the UK the statutory right to paid annual holiday from their first day of employment (EIRO 2001e).

In light of the UK's limited experience of statutory working time regulation, in addition to the ambiguity of many of the Directive's central provisions, the WTR have since been the subject of a number of legal challenges (Adnett and Hardy 2001: 121–3). This litigation has sought to determine the parameters of the UK Regulations and has led to the emergence of a body of case law from the British and European Courts. For example:

- in *R* v. *Attorney-General for Northern Ireland* ex parte *Burns* (1999), the High Court delivered an expansive ruling for the classification of night workers, establishing that an employee might be defined as a night worker even if they work between 9 pm and 7 am for only one week of every three-week shift cycle (Adnett and Hardy 2001: 121)
- in *Hill* v. *Howard Chappel* (2002), the Employment Appeal Tribunal (EAT) ruled that an employer is not permitted to deduct any overpaid holiday from an employee's final salary payment, unless a legally binding 'relevant agreement' authorises such a deduction (Lawzone 2002b).

With many commentators claiming that the Regulations still leave much to be determined by legal interpretation, further litigation is certain to follow (Lourie 1998: 24; Adnett and Hardy 2001). In particular, uncertainty remains in relation to who may be classified as a 'managing executive', the status of 'on-call' time in calculating the duration of a worker's working time, the rights of overseas workers and whether bank holidays are included within the four weeks' paid holiday entitlements (Lawzone 2000, 2002a).

Potentially, this enhanced involvement of the law in UK working time arrangements will have far-reaching consequences. As Bercusson has cogently argued, 'the upshot of the WTD is that the organisation of working time is no longer the exclusive managerial prerogative of the employer, but is a process of mutual accommodation, subject ultimately to adjudication' (Bercusson 1996: 332). Therefore, 'by lending statutory support to the principle of consultation and negotiation over hours of work', the Regulations have helped to 'establish clearly and more widely working time arrangements as a primary concern of workplace industrial relations' (EIRO 2000b: 4). Moreover, the annual Warwick Pay and Working Time Survey has shown that many employers expect the Regulations to have 'important implications in the near to medium-term future' (EIRO 2000b: 3). Elsewhere, the Regulations concerning night work and shift work threaten to have a notable impact on certain sectors, including printing and the NHS. With the Government still to transpose the HAD and sector-specific Directives, this degree of influence will undoubtedly increase.

Likewise, much will depend on the outcome of the Commission's review of the Article 18 provision that currently enables individual workers to voluntarily opt-out from the 48-hour weekly working limit. The Directive prescribes that this review is to be undertaken by 23 November 2003. Should the Commission recommend an end to this provision, it could be removed by a qualified majority vote within the Council. As Britain is the only member state to have exercised this general exemption, and because the UK has the highest average weekly working hours for full-time workers in the UK, it is widely expected that the Commission will recommend its discontinuation (EIRO 2002b). With the future of the individual opt-out in doubt, the CBI is actively campaigning for its retention. The CBI has recently claimed that the individual opt-out is a 'core element of the UK's flexible labour market' and is 'one of the key factors behind the success of the UK economy and our low levels of unemployment' (CBI 2003: 1, 6). By contrast the TUC has urged the Government not to seek an extension of the current individual opt-out, in light of the UK's continuing 'long-hours culture' (TUC 2002).

Nevertheless, given the flexible and minimalist way in which the Regulations were framed, the practical consequences within firms have, to date, proved limited. Research sponsored by the DTI revealed that the majority of companies have encountered few problems complying with the Regulations (Neathey and Arrowsmith 2001). This is largely because the standards demanded by the Regulations have proved close to existing patterns of working time (Goss and Adam-Smith 2001: 198). As Neathey and Arrowsmith (2001) summarise:

- 'in most organisations, existing holiday entitlements for employees were in excess of the new statutory minimum' (Neathey and Arrowsmith 2001: 47)
- 'only a small number of organisations were exceeding the night-work limits prior to the Regulations' (Neathey and Arrowsmith 2001: 53)
- there is little evidence to suggest 'that these [health assessments] had resulted in workers being moved away from night work' (Neathey and Arrowsmith 2001: 72).

Overall, although some organisations have used the Regulations to launch a major review of their existing working time practices, most employers have sought to exploit the individual opt-outs, derogations and exemptions provided by the Regulations, in order to minimise the overall impact of the new legislation. This has been most notable in relation to the general exemption from the 48-hour weekly working limit. A 2001 CBI survey reported that an estimated 47% of companies have used opt-outs for some groups of workers, a figure which rises to 71% for larger companies with between 500 and 5000 employees (EIRO 2002b). Consequently, long hours continue to form a prominent feature of the British labour market while the Directive has proved to be 'a matter of little concern for most employers and their workers' (EIRO, May 2001f).

Implementing the Employee Participation Directives

By encouraging companies that fall under the scope of the EWCD to conclude voluntary 'Article 13' agreements, a crucial role in implementing the Directive's requirements is fulfilled by independent company agreements. As such, the Regulations do not apply to those undertakings that had concluded agreements for the transnational information and consultation of their entire EEA workforce prior to the Directive's implementation deadline (DTI 1999b).[21] However, statutory transposition of the EWCD has still been required to give legal effect to some important provisions (Carley and Hall 2000: 122). The Labour Government has fulfilled this function through the Transnational Information and Consultation of Employees Regulations 1999. Contrary to the Conservative Governments' hostile approach towards implementing the 'first wave' employee participation Directives, the new Labour Government has both facilitated and welcomed the extension of the EWCD to the UK. Under Labour, the DTI (1999c) claimed that the EWCD simply established certain 'sensible minimum standards for informing and consulting at the European level'. Nevertheless, by 'extending statutory rights to information and consultation and providing for standing works-council-type bodies', the Regulations do 'represent a further landmark in the "Europeanisation" of UK labour law' (Carley and Hall 2000: 103).

In accordance with the requirements of the Directive, the 1999 Regulations are primarily concerned with establishing:

- the procedures for selecting 'special negotiating body' (SNB) and statutory EWC members
- the status and enforcement of agreements
- the rules on withholding confidential information
- the procedures for establishing a statutory EWC.

Each of these has raised challenges and opportunities for the British industrial relations system. For example, whereas other member states were easily able to comply with the EWCD by using existing domestic representational structures, the UK's 'representation gap' forced the Government to introduce further 'issue-specific' procedures for electing or appointing national members of SNBs or statutory EWCs (Carley and Hall 2000: 123).

As collective agreements are not legally binding under UK law, the status of the three types of agreements that may be concluded in accordance with the Directive has raised a number of complex and contradictory responses. Firstly, in formulating the Regulations, it was the Government's view that pre-existing voluntary 'Article 13' agreements *do* constitute a form of collective agreement and are therefore not automatically binding on the parties concerned. As the Directive does not explicitly require 'Article 13' agreements to be binding, 'the Government has chosen not to elaborate on this point' (DTI 1999c: point 8). Instead the Regulations allow this feature of Britain's 'voluntarist' tradition to be preserved, by leaving it to the negotiators themselves to determine the legal status of the agreement and the arrangements for dispute resolution. By contrast, it was clear that statutory EWC agreements concluded in accordance with the Directive's subsidiary requirements and the Schedule to the Regulations *must* be legally binding. This required the introduction of new procedures to enable statutory agreements to be enforced and disputes to be resolved. Lastly, however, the status of 'Article 6' agreements negotiated pursuant to the Regulations was more ambiguous. A number of respondents to the Government's public consultation argued that these agreements would constitute a collective agreement under UK law and should therefore not be legally binding. Irrespective of these claims, the Government concluded that these EWC agreements implement obligations imposed by a Council Directive and must be enforceable (DTI 1999c). Consequently, the Regulations have introduced what are seen as a relatively complex series of enforcement procedures conducted through the Employment Appeal Tribunal (EAT) and Central Arbitration Committee (CAC).

The EAT hears disputes about the non-establishment of an EWC and the operation of existing EWC agreements, and has the power to impose a financial penalty on management of up to £75 000 but lacks the capacity to suspend or overturn those management decisions taken in breach of an EWC agreement as exists in other member states (EIRO 1999e). The CAC hears disputes relating to whether an undertaking is subject to the Directive/Regulations, the SNB selection procedures leading to the establishment of an EWC, and whether confidentiality clauses have been breached (DTI 1999c). Overall, the EAT and CAC represent the institutional compromise between the Government's need to fulfil the terms of the directive, maintain the voluntarist nature of the UK system and see disputes resolved 'as quickly and flexibly as possible' (DTI 1999d).

Complications have also arisen over the protection of confidential business information (Carley and Hall 2000: 118). In close accordance with the minimum terms of the Directive, the Regulations prevent SNB/EWC members from disclosing any information that management has required must be held in confidence. Central management are also permitted to withhold any information that, according to 'objective criteria', would seriously harm or prove prejudicial to the functioning of the company. However, the Regulations do not establish what constitutes 'objective criteria' for the withholding of information. Instead, the Government envisaged 'that the test of serious harm or prejudice will have to be judged on a case-by-case basis in the light of all relevant circumstances' (Carley and Hall 2000: 119). Significantly, the regulations rely on civil, not criminal, remedies for breaches of confidentiality (EIRO 2000b).

Overall, the introduction of new statutory rights to information and consultation could transform a number of core principles within the UK's 'voluntarist' system of industrial relations. However, the Labour Government, by transposing the EWC directive in a minimalist fashion and fully exploiting the flexibility provided by the Directive, helped to mitigate the practical consequences of this fundamental legal change. Accordingly, there is no evidence that the Government 'gold-plated' any of the directive's provisions, and the regulations have generated relatively little controversy compared with the intensity of managerial opposition to the Directive in the run-up to its adoption (Carley and Hall 2000: 122–3).

Lastly, although the Government has yet to finalise its transposition legislation for the EU Directive on national information and consultation rules ahead of the March 2005 deadline, this legislation also stands to have a significant formal impact on British industrial relations (EIRO 2000a: 8). However, the Government has already indicated that it will adopt a flexible approach towards implementing the Directive, along broadly similar lines to the 1999 Transnational Information and Consultation of Employees Regulations (DTI 2003). Thus, one would expect to see a similar pattern of slow, small-scale adaptations that have the potential to significantly alter issue-specific procedures for the selection of employee representatives and pressure the current 'representation gap' in British industrial relations, but is unlikely to produce a large-scale shift in the basic voluntaristic nature of UK industrial relations.

Conclusion

The regulation of the European labour market to secure a body of statutory rights for employee participation and employment protection has proved to be one of the most acrimonious of EU 'social' policies, particularly in the UK. During the 'first wave' of policy activism, stretching from the mid-1970s to the early 1980s, many of the Commission's harmonising and ambitious proposals were obstructed by the British veto, for a combination of ideological and practical reasons. The second wave of legislation was more successful due to a more flexible and limited Commission approach (Streeck 1998: 436) and the growing use of QMV to surmount the British veto.

However, even though the EU *has* now adopted a significant body of labour law it 'cannot be presented as either a coherent, unitary or complete system of EC regulation' (Szyszczak 2000b: 164), and only regulates discrete aspects of the employment relationship. Consequently, many core areas of British industrial relations, including wages, collective bargaining and strikes, have remained untouched by the reach of EU labour law. In the areas where the EU *has* been able to legislate, these limitations have ensured that the legal rights and protections provided have been established at a relatively low level. Therefore, with the EU heavily restricted in the volume and form of labour law it can produce, many of the recent legislative developments in British labour market policy have been the result of a nationally constructed agenda. Although this agenda has included the extension of statutory regulation and a greater acceptance of partnership approaches – both features that are more prevalent within the 'continental' system of industrial relations – many of these changes are attributable to the Labour Government's desire to reconfigure aspects of the British labour market, rather than the existence of any formal adaptational pressure exerted by EU Directives.

This distinct pattern of integration over the last 30 years has contributed to the *partial* Europeanisation of British labour market policy. Despite the numerous limitations experienced in the integration process, where the EU *has* established a body of European labour law, its impact on UK labour market policy has often been significant. In adapting to the requirements of the EU labour market Directives, the law has extended ever further into Britain's 'voluntarist' system of industrial relations. Today, as a result of European and national factors, the law 'shapes UK industrial relations in a way that would have been inconceivable even in the recent past' (McKay 2001: 285). Despite attempts by the Conservative Government to limit the degree of domestic policy change imposed by the 'first wave' Directives, the rulings of the European Court have served as a powerful force of vertical Europeanisation. These rulings ultimately forced a reluctant Conservative Government to amend its initial transposition legislation for the Directives on acquired rights and collective redundancies. Even though doubts remained as to how effectively these changes brought Britain's legislation into line with the European requirements, the new *ad hoc* procedures for selecting employee representatives in the absence of a recognised trade union have represented a fundamental procedural change in British industrial relations.

More recently, under the Blair Government, the relationship between Britain and EU labour law has developed along a more consensual path. At an ideological level this reflects the fact that Labour has been more predisposed to the extension of workplace rights than its Conservative predecessor. However, on a practical level it is also an indication of the Government's acceptance of the increasingly flexible provisions of the 'second wave' of European legislation. In implementing the WTD and EWCD, the Blair Government fully exploited the derogations, exemptions and general flexibilities provided, as it attempted to balance the rights of employees with those of the employer and labour market efficiency. The Blair Government has outlined a similarly flexible approach towards implementing the 2002 national information and consultation directive. This demonstrates that although 'social justice may be an important consideration in "Third Way" industrial relations ... it is clearly not the only concern' (Undy 1999: 332).

By requiring the extension of statutory regulation into further areas of the British labour market, EU labour law has reconfigured important elements of Britain's 'voluntarist' industrial relations system. However, in so doing, a variety of national factors have prevented EU labour law from producing a strong body of individual and collective rights for British workers. This form of interactive partial Europeanisation produced a series of procedural changes in British industrial relations, rather than a substantive extension of workplace rights and protections. Although one may question the individual and cumulative merits of these directives, this pattern of influence clearly does not amount to the EU 'Superstate' doomsday scenario once widely predicted by the Conservative Governments of Thatcher and Major and elements of the British business community. It is possible that the impact of EU labour law could prove to be more significant in the medium to long term, particularly in regard to legal implications and developments. However, in the short term the window of opportunity for further European labour law remains narrow.

Final point: the EU–UK labour policy relationship – does the Labour Party matter?

As seen throughout this chapter, the adoption of the EU's labour law Directives has required the introduction of important changes to Britain's labour market policy in some areas and left others untouched. Obviously, these uneven developments have occurred in a changing national political context. The most obvious and significant change was the election of Tony Blair's Labour Government in 1997. How has Labour affected the EU-induced changes in UK labour market policy?

A leading policy objective of the new Blair Government was the introduction of a package of 'third way' reforms designed to modernise the British labour market. This agenda sought to promote the 'dynamic relationship between *fairness* and *efficiency*' (emphasis added) (The Labour Party 1997b). Here, efficiency within the labour market was deemed necessary to enhance UK competitiveness and 'generate prosperity for the country'. However, fairness within the labour market is seen as important 'because people at work deserve to be treated decently, but also because workers perform better when they are' (DTI 1998: 2.12). In this way fairness and efficiency are 'wholly compatible'. In his foreword to the influential 1998 White Paper: *Fairness At Work*, Tony Blair stated that these reforms constituted a new 'industrial relations settlement' for the UK. And while much of this 'settlement' was based upon the flexible implementation of the 'second wave' labour law Directives, it has also featured a body of nationally inspired 'reforms' centred around three main principles.

Firstly, in spite of Labour's commitment to social partnership, this 'settlement' included the retention of most of the restrictions on trade unions introduced by the Conservatives during the 1980s and early 1990s. As Labour's 1997 business manifesto explained:

> *The existing laws on industrial action, picketing and ballots will all remain unchanged. Every employee should be free to join or not join a trade union. We will not impose trade unions on employees or return to the closed shop* (Labour Party 1997b).

Secondly, it featured a number of initiatives designed to improve education and training in the British labour market, as a means to promote economic competitiveness, employment and greater social inclusion (EIRO 1997a). Thirdly, this 'settlement' sought to put in place a framework of statutory minimum employment rights to ensure the fair treatment of employees in the workplace. This included new and enhanced rights for individuals, in addition to a package of new collective rights. In the 1998 White Paper Blair argued:

> *Even after the changes we propose, Britain will have the most lightly regulated market of any leading economy in the world. But it cannot be just to deny British citizens basic canons of fairness ... that are a matter of course elsewhere* (DTI 1998).

These three principles resulted in a host of policy developments from new rights against unfair dismissal to new representation rights that were designed to provide new minimalist labour rights to workers and maintain the fundamentally market-oriented and voluntarist nature of the UK industrial relations system. Two examples highlight this balance particularly well. First, the Employment Relations Act 1999, which contained much of the 'Fairness at work' legislation, introduced a statutory procedure through which independent trade unions can seek recognition from employers for purposes of collective bargaining in relation to pay, hours and holidays (EIRO 1999c). Traditionally, the recognition of trade unions in the UK has been a voluntary matter for employers; the only previous statutory procedures under the Industrial Relations Act 1971 proved 'controversial and short-lived'. Although the 1999 Act seeks to encourage *voluntary* agreements, where a union claim for recognition cannot be resolved with the employer, the union is permitted to refer the matter to the CAC. The Act also establishes legal procedures for the de-recognition of unions, and protections for workers against detriment or dismissal for exercising their rights (EIRO 2000d). Although the long-term significance of these procedures remains to be seen, it is widely felt this measure could go some way to addressing the 'representation gap' in UK industrial relations, a gap that has caused serious problems for UK compliance with a number of European labour law Directives.

A second key Labour policy was the introduction of a national minimum wage in 1999,[22] based on the recommendations of the Low Pay Commission. Originally set in April 1999 at £3.60 for adults and £3.00 for those aged 18–21 years, it was estimated it benefited 1.9 million employees (8.3% of the workforce), particularly female workers and part-time workers of both sexes. The policy brought the UK into line with every other modern industrial country and represented a radical departure for British labour market policy. The UK did have some previous experience of statutory wage setting through the wages councils; however, this system had not provided universal coverage and had been progressively dismantled by the Conservatives during the 1980s and

1990s. At the time of their abolition in 1993, the wages councils had set minimum wage levels for some 2.5 million workers, their influence having fallen from a peak of 3.5 million workers in 1953 (EIRO, April 1999b). However, in the party's manifesto for the 1997 general election, Labour argued:

> *There should be a statutory level beneath which pay should not fall – with the minimum wage decided not on the basis of a rigid formula but according to the economic circumstances at the time ... Introduced sensibly the minimum wage will remove the worst excesses of low pay (and be of particular benefit to women), while cutting some of the massive £4 billion benefits bill by which the tax payer subsidies companies that pay very low wages* (The Labour Party 1997a).

Here again, we see the willingness of Labour to accept new minimalist standards without fundamentally altering the basic voluntarist structure. These changes do matter, particularly to those at the bottom of the pay scale, but do not represent a fundamental system shift. This can be visualised using the complexity perspective in Figure 7.1.

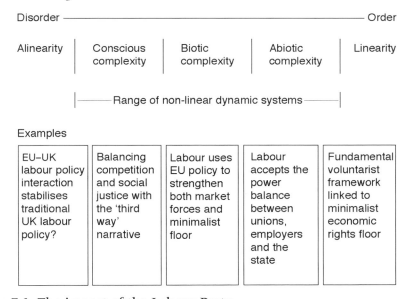

Figure 7.1 **The impact of the Labour Party.**

Notes

1 Directive 75/129/EEC.
2 Directive 77/187/EEC.
3 Directive 98/50/EC (OJ 1998 L201/88).
4 Directive 80/987/EEC.
5 Sections 122–127 of the Employment Protection (Consolidation) Act 1978.
6 The CRD was implemented in the UK by the Employment Protection Act 1974 (Part IV) and is currently contained under the Trade Union and Labour Relations (Consolidation) Act 1992 (Section 188–198). Under the UK Regulations a collective

redundancy is defined as one where, over a 90-day period, 20 or more employees are to be dismissed at one establishment.

7 Collective Redundancies Directive, Article 2.1; Acquired Rights Directive. Article 6.2.
8 Section 11 of the Employment Protection Act 1975.
9 Case C-382/92 (1994) IRLR 392 and Case C-383/92 (1994) IRLR 412.
10 Directive 91/533/EC.
11 Directive 96/71/EC.
12 Directive 94/33/EC.
13 The Government abolished the prohibition of night work for women and children (Employment Act 1989), and lifted restrictions on Sunday working (Sunday Trading Act 1989).
14 New Article 138.
15 This was later modified by the 2000 Horizontal Amending Directive (Directive 2000/34/EC) that extended the Directive to cover 'non-mobile' workers in the sectors and others not covered by specific Social Partner agreements.
16 The EWCD has since been extended to cover the whole of the European Economic Area (Norway, Iceland and Liechtenstein).
17 Directive 2001/86/EC.
18 Britain and Ireland successfully negotiated an extended transition period for smaller companies, meaning the Directive will only become fully operational in the UK from 23 March 2008.
19 The Regulations also implement the provisions of the Young Workers' Directive that relates to the hours of work of young people aged over the minimum school leaving age, but under 18 years.
20 Case C-173/99 – *R* v. *Secretary of State for Trade and Industry*, ex parte *Broadcasting, Entertainment, Cinematograph and Theatre Union*.
21 For those undertakings covered by the original Directive, the deadline for concluding Article 13 agreements was 22 September 1996. For those undertakings brought within the legislation's scope by way of the Extension Directive, relevant company agreements had to be concluded by 15 December 1999. Although these provisions are contained under Article 3 of the Extension Directive, the term 'Article 13 agreement' has continued to be used.
22 The National Minimum Wage Act 1998 provided powers for the Government to adopt Regulations to implement the national minimum wage.

Chapter 8

Economic and monetary union: the future of the economic foundation of the UK welfare state

For many, the fate of the UK welfare state hinges much more on the economics of the EU than on particular social policy developments. Does the European Union (EU) enhance the British economy, thereby creating an economic foundation for sustainable UK welfare state activity? Or, does the EU's competitive pressures and free market orientation constrain and restrict UK welfare state development? Nowhere is this debate more fierce than in regard to the European Monetary Union (EMU) and whether the UK should be in or out of it. For pro-Europeans, EMU is merely the next step in a logical expansion of EU competencies, is necessary to enhance the functioning of internal markets and may lead to further European political and economic integration. Anti-Europeans fear the continual expansion of an EU 'superstate', regret the loss of national autonomy and bemoan the loss of the Pound, a potent British symbol. With the successful development of EMU after Maastricht and the launch of the Euro in 1999, the issue has deeply divided both British elites and the general population. Britain's relationship to the euro has been one of continual uncertainty, 'opt-outs', 'economic tests', deferred decisions and referenda.

But how can one assess the impact of EMU on the UK welfare state when the UK is not a member? To surmount this difficulty one must come to grips with the basic parameters of both EMU and British monetary and fiscal policy, explore how EMU has affected member states that are in the eurozone and study how the UK has been affected by not joining the euro. Following this, one can begin to speculate on the current and potential impacts of EMU on the economic and monetary policy foundations of the UK welfare state and capture some of the complex range of Europeanising dynamics EMU would exert should Britain opt to join the euro.

The quest for European Monetary Union

For centuries, control of the national currency has been synonymous with the power of the state and a symbol of national autonomy (Currie 1999: 4). However, plans to 'pool' monetary sovereignty and forge a monetary union have been a recurring feature of the EU's integration agenda, the first such initiative dating back to 1969. While attempts by sovereign nation-states to seek exchange rate stability through fixed-but-adjustable exchange rate regimes have been a recurring theme throughout recent history, most notably through the Gold Standard and Bretton Woods System, monetary union constitutes the irrevocable fixing of exchange rates and free movement of capital across national frontiers (Healey 2000: 20). Although not an essential requirement of monetary union, the Maastricht agreement demanded the replacement of national currencies with a single currency – the euro. Yet if a monetary union is to prove successful and durable it *does* require the introduction of a common monetary policy (Johnson 1996: xi). To fulfil this function the Maastricht Treaty provided for the creation of the European Central Bank (ECB).

Why have the majority of member states been willing to abandon national monetary autonomy and seek the creation of a single currency? This has been the result of a complex of economic and political factors. The economic advantages most often cited in favour of monetary union include:

- the elimination of nominal exchange rate fluctuations within the eurozone, thereby providing a stimulus to trade and investment
- the elimination of transaction costs on cross-border trade
- greater price transparency, which should lead to increased competition throughout the eurozone
- an independent ECB should lead to lower average inflation and lower rates of interest (Layard 2000: 57).

Although joining a single currency involves giving up unilateral control over national monetary policy, the value of an independent currency as a tool of macroeconomic adjustment is widely questioned in today's globalised economy (Currie 1999: 5). With global financial markets trading more than a trillion dollars per day, nations need to ensure that their independent national currency remains as attractive to hold as its competitors. In this context, there is an important distinction between *de jure* sovereignty – what a nation-state can formally achieve – and *de facto* autonomy – what is feasible (Hine 1998: 1–2; Heath 2000: 203–5). As Leon Brittan (2000: 67) argued, monetary policy autonomy was heavily constrained during the 1980s and 1990s 'because in practice, interest rates across much of Europe were heavily determined by what the Bundesbank did in Germany'. This hegemonic position held by Germany was the result of the attractiveness of the Deutschmark in the financial markets and meant weaker currencies had to sustain higher rates of interest to attract investors. To overcome this situation, the majority of member states agreed at Maastricht to 'pool' formal monetary sovereignty, to ensure monetary policy was formulated according to the conditions in all member states, 'and not skewed, as in the Bundesbank-led ERM [Exchange Rate Mechanism], towards those in just one member state' (Levitt and Lord 2000: 44).

At Maastricht the founding Treaty was amended to incorporate the basis of Delors' three-stage plan for EMU. This plan tightly defined the convergence criteria necessary prior to the launch of the single currency, and established the institutional and common policy arrangements for the conduct of monetary affairs in the future eurozone. This 'paradigmatic change' was largely facilitated by the emergence of a firm consensus about the fundamental principles of monetary policy among a relatively small community of central bank governors (Dyson and Featherstone 1999: 3). The Delors Report published in April 1989 and signed by all central bank governors, including the Governor of the Bank of England Robin Leigh-Pemberton, expressed the desirability of forging a monetary union based on the German model of independent central bank governance. Therefore, in stark contrast to most other EU policy areas, a small 'technocratic elite' was able to capture control of a core area of national policy (Radaelli 2001: 16).

However, while 11 member states were prepared to commit to an irreversible timetable for realising EMU at the Maastricht intergovernmental conference (IGC), the UK Conservative Government, mirroring similar debates over European monetary integration in the 1970s and 1980s, remained beset by serious economic and political misgivings over British participation in the project (Giordano and Persaud 1998: 159–62). Some Conservatives supported plans for EMU, often on the basis of 'one market, one money' logic; for others, EMU challenged many core principles of Conservatism including entrenched notions of nationhood and sovereignty (Dyson and Featherstone 1999: 535). However, given the strength of commitment to the single currency project from the other member states, the Conservative Government was forced to respond to an agenda not of their choosing. In this context John Major saw that his only realistic option at the Maastricht IGC in December 1991 was to negotiate an 'opt-out' for the British.

British monetary policy today

The Protocol negotiated by John Major at Maastricht stated that should the British Government inform the Council of its intention not to move to the third stage of EMU, the 'United Kingdom shall retain its powers in the field of monetary policy according to national law'.[1] As a result of the new Labour Government's decision to exercise this prerogative, British monetary policy remains subject to the terms of the new policy framework unveiled by Tony Blair's Government shortly after its accession to power in May 1997 (HM Treasury 1999b).

The primary objective of Britain's new monetary policy arrangements is to maintain price stability in order to achieve the Government's central macroeconomic objective of high and stable levels of growth and employment (HM Treasury 1999b: 1–5, 17). In order to achieve and maintain price stability, separate and unambiguous roles for the Government and the Monetary Policy Committee (MPC) of the Bank of England were created for the conduct of UK monetary policy, later formalised by the Bank of England Act 1998. Under these procedures, the Government, via the Treasury, establishes the objectives of monetary policy while the Bank ensures these objectives are met. The Treasury defines price stability through the setting of a symmetrical target inflation rate while the MPC sets interest rates, on the basis of a majority vote of its nine members, to achieve the Treasury's inflation target.

Central to the changes introduced under the new monetary policy framework was the Government's decision to grant the Bank of England operational independence in fulfilling its price stability mandate. The move reflected an emerging consensus amongst financial elites in advanced economies that independent experts, being 'unencumbered by short-term political pressures, are best able to make forward-looking decisions in the long-term interests of the economy' (HM Treasury 1999b: 2) and generate sustained price stability (Abbott 2000; Levitt and Lord 2000). In response to the obviously anti-democratic nature of this decision, Labour has gone to great lengths to ensure that high levels of openness, transparency and accountability have accompanied the granting of central bank independence (HM Treasury 1999b). For example, the MPC has to fulfil a raft of reporting obligations and despite its independence is still accountable for its performance to the Treasury Committee and the House of Lords Select Committee.

European Central Bank monetary policy: implications for the UK

For participating member states, EMU has radically reconfigured the structure of power in monetary policy, with responsibility having transferred from national to European level institutions (Featherstone 1999: 324; Radaelli 2001). At present, while the UK remains unaffected by formal obligations to the ECB, if Britain were to join the single currency, it too would be subject to this same process of transformation with responsibility for monetary policy transferring from the Treasury and Bank of England to the ECB and would constitute a significant Europeanisation of British economic policy. However, as will be shown, the implications of such a transformation would not be felt evenly across all dimensions of British monetary policy, thus again illustrating the complexity and contingency of (potential) Europeanising dynamics.

Although EMU exerts powerful forces of vertical Europeanisation, the implications of this change are lower for those member states with similar monetary policy regimes to the new ECB. Research has revealed that during the 1980s a number of countries adopted a new monetary policy regime in order to align themselves with the German Bundesbank – the hegemonic monetary system at the time and model for the subsequent ECB (Pochet 1999: 16). This convergence towards the German model of central bank governance, before the Maastricht Treaty indicates a form of horizontal Europeanisation, was inducing policy change in this direction in the decade prior to the Maastricht agreement (Dyson 2000: 649). Indeed these changes help explain why EMU was agreed at Maastricht, and reflect the 'diffusion of ideas and discourses about the notion of good policy' among a relatively small policy community (Radaelli 2001: 12).

These modifications to national monetary policy regimes in the run up to the changeover helped mitigate the potential difficulties of the transition to EMU for the majority of member states. In recent years Britain, too, has modified its monetary policy framework in the direction of the dominant German/ECB model, indicating that the UK has also been subject to a subtle yet powerful force of horizontal Europeanisation while remaining outside of EMU. This is a development which would ease Britain's transition to the single currency should the UK ultimately decide to join the euro. These changes have been most notable in respect of the Bank of England being granted operational independence, but also in the current rejection of devaluation in favour of inflation-targeting and long-term monetary stability (Pochet 1999: 16).

The primary responsibility of the ECB, like the Bank of England since the 1997 changes, is to maintain price stability, and although the ECB is also obliged to 'support the general economic policies of the Community', these actions must not compromise this primary objective.[2] Differences do exist between the mandates given to the respective banks, for while the MPC is presented with an explicit inflation target set by the Treasury, the ECB is free to formulate its own target for price stability. Therefore, if Britain were to join the single currency, although the degree of vertical Europeanisation encountered would be significant as well as the location of power, the core objectives of monetary policy would remain the same.

Another major implication of a common monetary policy is that Britain would lose the option of devaluation as a strategy for macroeconomic adjustment. Indeed, the ability for the Government to manipulate the exchange rate has historically been the foundation of an independent monetary policy. However, the effects of this potential loss of sovereignty under EMU would be mitigated by the fact the Bank of England is currently pursuing a monetary policy similar to the ECB; that is, one set in the medium term with a primary commitment to price stability, thereby eschewing such a short-term stabilisation role for monetary policy. Moreover, the long-term benefits of currency devaluation are increasingly open to question. Britain's own experience of devaluation has shown that the short-term benefits can be quickly eroded by higher inflation, it cannot address structural economic weaknesses, and it may ultimately undermine the credibility of the national currency (Crawford 1996: 334; Johnson 1996: 93). Therefore, in relation to the price stability mandate and the loss of the devaluation option, the impact for Britain of a Europeanised monetary policy would appear minimal.

For many, the greatest threat to UK economic independence and performance under EMU would be the loss of the ability to set interest rates unilaterally in accordance with the requirements of the national economy (Temperton 2001: 104). This loss of monetary policy independence would be moderated:

1 if the economic cycles in different eurozone countries coincided; and
2 if the ECB's monetary policy had the same effect in each country (Currie 1999: 9).

The convergence criteria in the years leading up to EMU were designed to fulfil these conditions and ensure the eurozone became an optimal currency area. Opinions differ as to how effectively the eurozone, with its current composition, is coping under a common monetary policy and interest rate. The EU Economy 2001 Review acknowledged that 'the lack of tailored monetary policy in individual euro-area member states increases the risk of pronounced financial cycles' (European Commission 2001b). These effects have proved particularly acute for Germany, where interest rates have been deemed too low, and Ireland, where by the halving of interest rates before joining the euro triggered a credit boom that has contributed to the economy overheating.

In Britain, similar concerns are not uncommon. As Sir Eddie George, the Governor of the Bank of England stated, 'certainly I see the one-size-fits all monetary policy as a disadvantage and a special risk. The same monetary policy is not optimal for every country at the same time' (*The Guardian*, 29 December

2001). These fears are exacerbated by evidence that the British economy, at present, does not meet the two conditions detailed above. Firstly, there is concern that Britain is more susceptible to asymmetric shocks than the core economies at the heart of the eurozone. Work undertaken by Phillipe Pochet to correlate the findings of a number of independent studies into the potential for asymmetric shocks reveals that Britain is consistently classified as a 'peripheral' country, where the risk of asymmetric shocks under EMU is seen to be greatest (Pochet 1999: 17–20). If the cycles of the British economy are not adequately aligned with those of the eurozone's core members, then the ECB's common interest rate, based on aggregate conditions throughout the eurozone, is likely to be set at a suboptimal level for British circumstances. Secondly, evidence of structural differences between Britain and continental Europe is also often used to demonstrate that Britain is more sensitive to interest rate changes than the core members. For example, the UK has a much higher level of household debt than other member states, meaning that a rise in interest rates may have a disproportionate effect on UK borrowers (*The Economist,* 28 March 1998; Giordano and Persaud 1998: 169).

Another complicating factor is the degree of central bank independence. Despite many similarities, the extent of the ECB's independence far surpasses that of the Bank of England and even the levels previously enjoyed by the German Bundesbank. As the European Parliament's Economic and Monetary Affairs Committee has argued:

> *The Statute of the ECB and the Maastricht Treaty take to new lengths the principle that a central bank should be independent. No other central bank – in any other political system – has been as independent* (European Parliament 1998).

As was shown when discussing the independence of the Bank of England, any decision to grant central bank autonomy must be accompanied by adequate procedures to ensure the bank remains accountable for the policies it conducts. Accountability is essential for any democratic system, yet in relation to the conduct of monetary policy, accountability can also help reinforce its credibility and performance without compromising independence (Levitt and Lord 2000: 225). In respect of Britain's possible future participation in EMU, it is the ECB's lack of transparency and accountability that has raised some of the greatest concerns. Indeed Featherstone (1999: 326) has argued 'nowhere is the problem of the EU's "democratic deficit" more pronounced than it is in the domain of EMU'.

There are some limits to the independence of the ECB. Though the minutes and voting records of the ECB remaining unpublished, the ECB is accountable to the Economic and Finance (ECOFIN) Council and European Parliament. Most notably, the president of the ECOFIN Council is permitted to attend meetings of the governing council of the ECB. While this is an important right, further efforts to make the ECB accountable to the Council have been resisted (Levitt and Lord 2000: 229–30). In this context, the European Parliament assumes an important role. Although the Parliament enjoys wide powers, they are relatively weak. In addition to hearing an annual report of the bank's activities delivered by the ECB President, the Parliament can also request explanations from the President and other ECB board members before the

Economic and Monetary Affairs Committee (EMAC). Furthermore, the Parliament has the right to be consulted on the appointment of the ECB president and other executive board members, while its approval is required under the assent procedure for most changes to the ECB Statute. These procedures may yet prove sufficient for the Council and Parliament to effectively hold the ECB to account. The Parliament has already actively sought to maximise its limited powers and it is widely acknowledged that it will take time for the necessary inter-institutional relationships to develop. However, it is clear that today, if the British Government wished to alter the independence of the Bank of England or change the MPC's policy mandate, it may do this through a simple Act of Parliament. Changing the ECB would be far harder.

Coordinating European fiscal policy

The extent to which national governments are required to coordinate their taxing and spending policies under monetary union has proved 'the most contentious issue of the entire EMU debate' (Gros and Thygesen 1998: 318). Given the loss of monetary policy as a tool for domestic macroeconomic management under EMU, greater responsibility falls on national budgetary policies as a means of adjustment to asymmetric shocks (HM Treasury 2001: 25). This is compounded by the fact that the EU currently lacks other traditional mechanisms for macroeconomic stabilisation, most notably a substantial budgetary role for regional transfers or a high degree of labour mobility. In this environment, a degree of fiscal coordination is widely deemed necessary to ensure that national budgetary policies complement the monetary strategy of the ECB and contribute to the EU's objectives of price stability, growth and employment.[3]

While there is broad acceptance that EMU requires some form of coordination to provide a suitable policy mix between monetary and fiscal policies, opinion is divided as to how this is best achieved. This is complicated by the role fiscal policy plays in social and redistribution policy as well as macroeconomic stabilisation policy (Gros and Thygesen 1998: 318; Levitt and Lord 2000: 145). The earlier Werner Plan for economic and monetary union advocated a new 'centre of decision for economic policy' to ensure a suitable policy mix between monetary, fiscal and social goals (Dyson and Featherstone 1999: 784). However, the later Delors Report, which formed the basis of the relevant Maastricht Treaty provisions, adopted an intergovernmental rule-based procedure centred around the ECOFIN Council, thereby removing the need for the centralisation of member states' economic policies at the European level. Consequently, while responsibility for monetary policy is transferred to a common supranational institution under stage three of EMU, budgetary policies remain under national control, subject to two complementary procedures: the Broad Economic Policy Guidelines (BEPGs) and the Stability and Growth Pact (SGP).

Current UK fiscal policy

As part of the overhaul of British macroeconomic management, the 1997 Labour Government introduced a new set of fiscal policy procedures to complement the changes made by the introduction of the new monetary policy framework. Consequently, the current fiscal policy objectives are:

- to ensure sound public finances and that intergenerational spending and taxation impact fairly both within and across generations
- to support monetary policy, where possible, by using automatic stabilisers and prudent fiscal alterations to stabilise demand (HM Treasury 1999a: 1).

To achieve these objectives, the Government has specified two fiscal rules:

- **the golden rule:** over the economic cycle, the Government will borrow only to invest and not to fund current spending
- **the sustainable investment rule:** public sector net debt as a proportion of gross domestic product (GDP) will be held over the economic cycle at a stable and prudent level (HM Treasury 1999a: 2).

Therefore, a core element of the UK's fiscal policy strategy is to pursue a sound and sustainable basis for public finances, but without limiting its ability to support monetary policy in cushioning the impact of the economic cycle (HM Treasury 2001: 9–12). The Government feels the primary way fiscal policy can smooth the path of the economy is through the full functioning of the automatic stabilisers. As such, public sector net borrowing (PSNB) is permitted to vary between years according to the economic cycle.

A number of procedures ensure that national monetary and fiscal policies combine to forge the distinctive UK policy mix. Firstly, the core objectives of monetary and fiscal policy are both currently set by the Government, meaning the two arms of policy may be mutually consistent and can work in a coordinated way to deliver economic stability (HM Treasury 2001: 9). Secondly, the process is conducted in the full view of the public and markets and with narrowly defined objectives. Likewise, the Code for Fiscal Stability requires the Treasury to place an emphasis on transparency by communicating its policy stance through the Budget, the pre-budget report and other supporting documents (HM Treasury 1999a: 29, 2001: 17). Thirdly, Treasury representation at the monthly Monetary Policy Committee (MPC) meetings ensures that the Committee is aware of fiscal policy developments. This combination of central government coordination and public openness are key to obtaining a reasonable and politically acceptable monetary and fiscal policy mix in the UK.

European procedures: general economic and detailed fiscal coordination

Under EMU, member states must coordinate many of their economic policies through multilateral surveillance procedures of the BEPGs. However, fiscal policies are much more constrained with specific rules for limiting national budgetary deficits and levels of debt through the Excessive Deficit Procedure (EDP),[4] and the Stability and Growth Pact (SGP).[5]

Whilst the negative effects of budgetary deficits are of primary concern, the EU has introduced procedures to coordinate a broad range of economic variables. The multilateral surveillance of national budgetary policies is therefore deemed necessary to ensure economic convergence between member states both inside and outside of the eurozone. Further, the BEPGs provide the framework for the definition of the overall macroeconomic policy objectives of the EU, seek to promote 'growth- and stability-oriented macroeconomic policies and comprehensive economic reforms of labour, product and capital markets' (Council of the European Union 2001a: 4) and contribute to the 'mutual reinforcement of economic and social policies' (Council of the European Union 2001a: 8). However, as shown below, in recent years the multilateral surveillance procedure has assumed an increasingly important role in the early identification and prevention of excessive deficits in accordance with the Stability Pact.[6]

The multilateral surveillance of national economic policies outlined under Article 99 of the Treaty is a soft regulatory form of governance of particular importance to the Community. It centres on an annual 'rolling process' of BEPGs issued by the Council, nationally submitted stability programmes (for countries participating in EMU), or convergence programmes (for non-participating member states), and a process of peer review undertaken by the Council.[7] Having evaluated the stability/convergence programmes in light of the Guidelines, the Council can issue Recommendations to both 'Ins' and 'Outs' (like Britain). These Recommendations, adopted by a qualified majority in ECOFIN, do not carry legal redress and rely solely on a process of 'naming and shaming' to induce national policy change.

Regarding fiscal policy coordination, the primary justification for constraints on national budgetary policies concerns the notion that budget deficits raise interest rates (Arestis and Sawyer 2000: 102). Although the extent of the spillover effect is contested, it is argued that fiscal expansion in one country can have external effects that drive up interest rates throughout the eurozone (Gros and Thygesen 1998: 320–6). Therefore, procedures for fiscal coordination are required to overcome the potential for profligate member states to 'free-ride' on the prudence of others. As was explained by Ireland's finance minister in 1996, 'if you have a joint bank account, it makes sense to put limits on the use of the cheque book' (*The Financial Times*, 21 May 2002).

Under Article 104, the Treaty states that member states shall avoid excessive government deficits. Significantly, as a result of the Protocol negotiated by the UK at Maastricht, this obligation does not apply to Britain unless it moves to stage three. Instead, Britain maintains its stage two obligation to '*endeavour* to avoid excessive government deficits' (emphasis added).[8] Under these rules, while the UK must comply with the peer review process of the BEPGs in respect of limits on national deficits, it will escape the Council's timed deficit reduction procedures and accompanying sanctions applicable to all eurozone members (Johnson 1996: 154).

For participating member states a separate Protocol established the reference values for the EDP as:

- 3% for the ratio of the planned or actual government deficit to GDP
- 60% for the ratio of government debt to GDP.

The EDP also established the procedures by which the Council may determine whether a member state has an excessive deficit, and the measures to be taken to rectify the situation. However, doubts were soon raised as to whether these measures were stringent enough to guarantee compliance. This led the German Government to propose a Pact to strengthen and clarify the EDP (Brunila *et al.* 2002: 5). The resultant Stability and Growth Pact enhances the original procedures by providing mechanisms 'both for prevention and deterrence', to ensure the 3% deficit limit is not breached (Council of the European Union 1997a).

The main preventative element of the Pact is a requirement that member states set medium-term budgetary targets that are 'close to balance or in surplus' in their annual stability or convergence programmes. The underlying philosophy behind the SGP is that:

> *Adherence to the objective of sound budgetary positions close to balance or in*
> *surplus will allow all member states to deal with normal cyclical fluctuations*
> *while keeping the government deficit within the reference value of 3% of GDP*
> (Council of the European Union 1997a).

To ensure this obligation is met, the multilateral surveillance of national budgetary positions assumes greater prominence under the SGP, as the Council seeks to prevent deficits from developing in the first place (Council of the European Union 1997b). A medium-term objective of a budget 'close to balance or in surplus' is therefore a core requirement of the BEPGs, and member states are required to express how they will meet this in their stability or convergence programmes. In recent years, member states have been required to move towards this budgetary position as soon as possible, and at the latest by 2004 (Council of the European Union 2002b; European Commission 2002a). The UK *is* currently subject to this system of multilateral surveillance and can receive Recommendations if the Commission detects slippage from the targets identified within the Guidelines (Brunila *et al.* 2002: 7).

The dissuasive element of the Pact is contained in a Council Regulation on speeding up and clarifying the EDP (Council of the European Union 1997c; Brunila *et al.* 2002: 7). It comprises an intergovernmental agreement which pre-commits member states to vote for sanctions, in the absence of 'exceptional circumstances', once a country has a deficit in excess of the 3% ceiling (Gros and Thygesen 1998: 343; Council of the European Union 1997c). Therefore, significantly, the assessment of whether a country has an excessive deficit is a political decision, determined by a qualified majority vote (QMV) within ECOFIN following a recommendation from the Commission, rather than occurring automatically after the 3% threshold has been breached. The SGP also elaborates on the timing and nature of sanctions should a country be found to have an excessive deficit. These complicated procedures are necessary because the Treaty explicitly excludes the Community's normal enforcement mechanisms through the European Court of Justice (ECJ) in this area (Gros and Thygesen 1998: 341). Again, in line with the preventative approach, a member state deemed to be nearing the upper deficit limit is first liable to receive an 'early warning' from the Council and be instructed to take remedial action to reduce the deficit. If this is unsuccessful and the 3% threshold is breached, the full procedure is activated and financial penalties may be imposed.

Fiscal policy coordination in practice: lessons from other member states

Overall, the Commission feels these procedures for fiscal coordination provide the Community with an appropriate policy mix and lower interest rates. As the Economic and Monetary Affairs Commissioner Pedro Solbes argued:

> *I think the existence of the pact gives the ECB more margin for manoeuvre and provides more certainty about eurozone budgetary policy* (in FT.com, 9 September 2001).

However, in the few years these procedures have been operating, they have aroused a significant degree of controversy both within the academic community and among the member states. For example, a frequently voiced concern is that a strict and inflexible interpretation of the SGP could prove pro-cyclical. Unless member states achieve a budget 'close to balance or in surplus' before the next economic downturn, then the SGP, if strictly interpreted and applied, would prevent the full functioning of the automatic stabilisers in softening the slowdown. This could require governments to raise taxes and cut expenditure to avoid breaching the deficit limit. Such a response would serve to exacerbate 'the recessionary tendency of the economy'. This effect would be amplified if the financial sanctions within the Pact were invoked (Eichengreen 2000: 88; Levitt and Lord 2000: 155) and create a 'deflationary bias' (Arestis and Sawyer 2000: 106). Paradoxically, as the multilateral surveillance of national policies under the BEPGs relies solely on peer pressure to induce domestic policy change, others are concerned that the procedures are too weak to constrain profligate countries, arguing that member states will be unwilling to pass negative judgements on one another or use the sanctions provided under the SGP (Levitt and Lord 2000: 214). Obviously, as these procedures for fiscal coordination have been functioning for a relatively short time, reaching firm conclusions as to their impact on national budgetary policies is a difficult undertaking (Fatás and Mihov 2000).

But what would happen to UK fiscal policy if the UK did join the euro? One way of looking at this is to see how other member states have been affected. An interesting case is the fate of the booming Irish economy. In February 2001 Ireland became the first member state to receive a formal reprimand from the ECOFIN Council. By pledging to boost spending and cut taxes in the context of existing inflationary pressures, the Council feared these measures could fan the flames of an already overheating Irish economy. Consequently, the ECOFIN Council recommended that the Irish take countervailing budgetary measures in the ensuing fiscal year. In response, Ireland's finance minister Charlie McCreevy was scathing of the formal reprimand arguing, with some justification, that Ireland was enjoying high levels of economic growth and had a budget *surplus* of 4.7%. Furthermore, as the Irish economy represented just 1% of the combined GDP of the eurozone, these measures posed no threat to the overall stability of the European economy (*Sunday Times* 18 February 2001). While there was some sympathy for the Irish situation, the Commission and Council felt that invoking the reprimand was necessary to demonstrate that they would use their power to make sure that all member states would abide by the rules for budgetary prudence. However, McCreevy's insistence that he would not amend his budgetary plans revealed that the system ultimately relies on peer pressure to induce domestic policy change. Unless the member state concerned has breached the 3% deficit ceiling, the Council is unable to exert stronger sanctions. In this instance the adaptational pressure exerted on the Irish Government proved insufficient to induce such change.

A different and more threatening development, excessive deficits, is found in the cases of Portugal, France and Germany. Portugal became the first member state to smash through the 3% ceiling by registering a budget deficit of 4.1% for 2001. In January 2003 Germany, the architect of the Stability and Growth Pact, was formally judged to have a general government deficit of 3.8% of GDP, while France became the third eurozone member to breach the budget deficit limit in June 2003 by registering a figure of 3.4% of GDP. All three countries received formal Council Recommendations demanding the national authorities put an end to the excessive deficit situation as rapidly as possible.

Clearly neither the prospect of strong financial sanctions nor the current procedures for multilateral surveillance have been able to prevent these countries from exceeding the 3% deficit ceiling. Consequently, in 2002, in an attempt to salvage the Pact, the Commission announced a package of reforms designed to improve the interpretation and implementation of the SGP (European Commission 2002e) and agreed to allow member states an extra two years beyond the original 2004 deadline to get their public finances close to balance or in surplus (*The Independent*, 23 October 2002). While the core budget requirements of the Pact remain unchanged, the reforms aim to inject more flexibility into how it is interpreted. Most significantly this includes:

- defining the 'close to balance or in surplus' requirement in underlying terms, thereby taking account of the economic cycle
- attaching greater importance to government debt levels in the budgetary surveillance process to improve the sustainability of public finances.

Interestingly, these reforms bring the EU's fiscal policy framework broadly in line with the British Treasury's 'golden rule' and 'sustainable investment rule'. As such, the changes should satisfy the UK's long-standing demands for a more 'prudent interpretation' of the Stability Pact (HM Treasury 2002b: 3).

In response to the Council's formal Opinion and Recommendation, Portugal has successfully reduced its general government deficit below 3% of GDP in 2002, in spite of weaker than anticipated growth. By contrast, although the German and French Governments remain formally committed to reducing their budget deficits, their progress has been limited. The European Commission's Report on the implementation of the 2002 BEPGs claimed Germany had implemented no new measures to ensure the 3% deficit would not be breached. Consequently, with economic growth also lower than previously forecast, Germany looks set to exceed the deficit limit again in 2003 and will find it difficult to reach the new medium-term budget target (close to balance by 2006) (European Commission 2003: 59). In late June 2003 the Pact faced a further challenge when Germany announced tax cuts worth €15.5 billion to stimulate growth in the country's stagnating economy. This announcement was welcomed in Paris where a senior French official claimed the move would make it easier for President Chirac to honour his year-old electoral pledge to cut taxes, despite France's widening deficit (FT.com, 30 June 2003). Yet significant tax cuts of this nature could put even greater pressure on Germany's already sizeable budget deficit. In this context many economists now claim the Pact has effectively been suspended until growth returns.

Such uncertainty means it is particularly difficult to predict the impact of these procedures on UK fiscal policy should Britain join the single currency. Nevertheless, one generality does seem apparent: being a larger member state seems to bring with it a greater degree of flexibility in applying the rules of EMU. However, the exact nature of that flexibility will clearly depend on the particular situation.

Fiscal policy coordination in practice: the impact on the UK

In the UK case, the fiscal policy framework unveiled by Labour in 1997 shares broad similarities with the annual BEPGs. The 'sustainable investment rule' provides for a prudent approach to debt accumulation, while both the British and European frameworks eschew a role for discretionary fiscal adjustments, preferring instead to allow the automatic stabilisers to smooth the path of the economy. However, Labour has repeatedly emphasised that, in line with its 'golden rule', the fiscal stance should be set over the entire economic cycle to allow surpluses in the current budget to offset weaker periods of growth. 'Attempting to balance the budget at all times would significantly increase swings in output over the economic cycle, damaging economic stability' (HM Treasury 2001: 10). As such the Labour Government has consistently demanded a more flexible interpretation of the SGP to relate to cyclically adjusted budget positions.

Although as an 'Out' the UK cannot face sanctions under the SGP, Britain is subject to the annual process of BEPGs and must submit a detailed convergence programme for the purposes of peer review. In recent years, the Government's projections within the UK's convergence programmes show that Britain comfortably meets the reference value for general government gross debt (60% of GDP), and to a lesser extent the reference value for general net borrowing (3% of GDP). Levels of gross debt are predicted to fall from 43.1% of GDP in 1999–2000 to 38.8% of GDP by 2003–2004 (HM Treasury 2002b: 28). However, Britain is unique among member states in actively choosing to move from a budget surplus to a deficit over the projection period, to fund improvements in priority public services (HM Treasury 2001: 30). The UK Convergence Programme 2000 projected that a budget surplus of 1.7% would move to a small deficit, stabilising at around 1% of GDP in the remaining years of the Programme to 2006–2007 (HM Treasury 2000). As a result of the global economic slowdown, these figures have since been revised with the UK's nominal budget deficit rising to 2.2% in 2003–2004, before stabilising at 1.6% to 2007–2008 (Council of the European Union 2003). The Government claims these projections are 'consistent with a broad interpretation of the SGP, which takes into account the economic cycle, sustainability and the important role of public investment' (HM Treasury 2001: 30).

Despite these broadly favourable figures, the Community's surveillance of Britain's budgetary policies generated a degree of controversy during 2001 and 2002. In response to the UK's Convergence Programme for 2000 (HM Treasury 2000), the Commission issued a favourable report commending Britain's efforts to raise employment and productivity levels and stated that Britain was well within the Maastricht criteria for joining the single currency (*The Sunday Times*, 18 February 2001). However, the report expressed a modest degree of concern about the extent of Britain's expansionary investment plans as they ran contrary to the BEPG's requirement for a budget of 'close to balance or in surplus'. Yet ultimately, the subsequent BEPGs for 2001 concluded the extra loosening was 'unlikely to compromise economic stability' (Council of the European Union 2001a: 67). This moderate criticism, within a broadly favourable report, elicited a fierce response from the Chancellor. In bellicose terms he argued that the budgetary plans met his 'golden rule' of fiscal policy, allowing the Government to borrow to invest in public services and were 'prudent, cautious and fiscally sound', adding these were 'the right things to do for British society and the economy' (*The Guardian*, 13 February 2001; *The Times*, 12 February 2001). As a result, Gordon Brown insisted his budgetary plans were non-negotiable.

This pattern of events was repeated during 2002. Whereas the BEPGs for 2002 again recommended that Britain should aim for a budget of 'close to balance or in surplus' by 2004, the UK's projected budget deficit equalled 1.1% of GDP. The Treasury calculated that to cut the deficit to zero would require spending cuts or tax increases totalling £10–11 billion. This led Gordon Brown to respond in forceful terms:

> *I certainly don't approve of a recommendation that would in effect ask us to cut £10bn from our very necessary spending on public services like health and transport* (FT.com, 10 February 2002).

However, to claim this is what the economic guidelines had actually stipulated is a 'cynical distortion of its view' (FT.com, 14 February 2002). The report primarily praises the UK, commending the projected fall in gross debt and stating that the UK is 'in a good position to meet the consequences of an ageing population' (European Commission 2002a: 65).

Therefore, to date, the Community's multilateral surveillance of Britain's budgetary policies has not led to significant changes in the UK's fiscal plans. However, as the Government's fiscal policy strategy has broadly coincided with the policy requirements of the BEPGs, the degree of policy adaptation required in Britain has been low. Gordon Brown's belligerent response to the two rounds of Guidelines can be seen as being for domestic consumption as he attempted to assert his authority on a larger European stage. This would not be the first time UK politicians have invented a fight with Europe from which they can proceed to claim victory. More importantly, this episode demonstrates that the peer review process is not a simple elite bargaining process, but plays out on a number of national and European political arenas.

Will EMU lead to a political union that undermines welfare?

Despite attempts by the UK Government to portray the single currency solely as an economic issue, the EMU project cannot easily be disentangled from the broader political dimension of European integration. For example, the Maastricht agreement that created EMU was also aimed at binding a reunified Germany into an EU framework. For other countries, the opportunity to participate in all decision-making processes at the European level provided a primary motivation for joining EMU (Pochet 1999: 20; de Schoutheete 2001). In this broader political context it is easy for both supporters and opponents of EMU to portray the project as a step on the road towards a broader 'political union' and an eventual federal state.

Although 'a single currency neither makes, nor requires a single state' (Smith 1998), many feel that for EMU to function effectively, the EU will be required to develop further state-like characteristics through a greater 'pooling' of sovereignty across a range of policy areas. Indeed if EMU and the euro do under-perform, demands for further integration are likely to intensify (Minford 2000: 78; FT.com, 20 May 2002). From a welfare state perspective, many observers have been concerned that if EMU did push the member states into deeper levels of integration then national social policies and provision would suffer. Three areas in particular are likely to see growing pressures for greater integration: fiscal policy, tax policy, and overall economic policy mix.

Fiscal federalism

If EMU is to be successful, other forms of adjustment to asymmetric shocks must compensate for the loss of monetary policy independence and constraints on national budgetary policies. In most modern federal states this stabilisation function is performed in part by the automatic contracyclical effect of the federal budget, as resources from faster growing regions are transferred to areas experiencing an economic downturn. Likewise federal budgets can also actively direct the redistribution of resources from richer to poorer areas through a system of inter-regional transfers aimed at the equalisation of standards of living. These stabilisation and redistribution functions of federal tax and social security regimes form the macroeconomic strategy of fiscal federalism.

The 1977 MacDougall Report argued that under EMU the Community would require a system of fiscal federalism to offset asymmetric shocks. It estimated the EC budget would need to increase to 5% of total GDP to fulfil this task (Eichengreen 2000: 87). While this figure remained far smaller than for most federal states, where budgets typically range between 20% and 40% of GDP, this would have represented a sizeable increase for the Community. However, by the time of the Delors' Report, fiscal federalism had been rejected in favour of mechanisms for fiscal policy coordination. As a result, the current EU budget does not serve an automatic contracyclical function as it is funded directly by member state contributions rather than through direct taxation on individuals and firms. Nor does it incorporate a 'federal' social security system (Arestis and Sawyer 2000: 101–2; Levitt and Lord 2000: 156–7). With the EU's entire budget currently accounting for only 1.27% of Community GDP, and half of this automatically devoted to the Common Agricultural Policy, the capacity for discretionary redistributive transfers through the Structural and Cohesion Funds remains relatively small. Furthermore, the Treaty requires that the Community's annual budget must balance. For these reasons, the current budget is poorly structured to fulfil an automatic pan-European stabilisation function, and too small to serve a significant role in inter-regional redistribution.

If the Community were to develop a system of fiscal federalism, significant reform would need to be undertaken both in terms of the size and structure of current funding arrangements. Although a number of economists have advocated the development of such a system (Gros and Thygesen 1998; Tondl 2000; MacDougall 2001), from a political perspective the significant constitutional reform that a system of fiscal federalism would require makes such a development a remote possibility (Eichengreen 2000: 97; Tondl 2000: 256). With a process of fiscal consolidation underway at the *national* level, initially through the convergence criteria and followed by the procedures for economic policy coordination, member states currently appear unprepared to sanction a major increase in fiscal transfers at the European level (Crouch 2000a: 22; Buti *et al.* 2003: 28). Furthermore, the Community arguably still lacks sufficient levels of social and political cohesion for a federal system of this nature to operate. Consequently, the issue has not featured as a serious proposition on the EU's current political agenda.

Tax harmonisation

While the EU has previously sought and attained a high degree of indirect tax harmonisation (European Commission 2001a), the launch of EMU has generated demands for further tax harmonisation. For example, in the late 1990s the former German finance minister Oskar Lafontaine frequently campaigned for greater tax harmonisation, while in 2001 the French Prime Minister Lionel Jospin claimed that 'ultimately the corporate tax system as a whole will have to be harmonised' (*The Times,* 29 May 2001). As taxation is widely seen as a core sovereign function of the nation-state, these demands have proved extremely controversial in the UK and are often given significant credence by Eurosceptic commentators (Redwood 2000: 219). Although the Labour Government accepts the need for greater coordination to 'tackle unfair tax practices, promote fair tax competition, and fight tax abuse and evasion directly', it views taxation as a matter for member states and opposes further tax harmonisation (HM Treasury 2002b: 33–4).

Following the introduction of the single currency, the need for domestic tax systems to contribute to the Lisbon objectives of growth and employment is heightened, as suboptimal economic performances will be externalised and felt throughout the entire eurozone. Furthermore, the euro will also reveal more clearly differences in the taxation regimes of member states, with investment likely to flow to the most favourable environment (Brittan 2000: 76). However, in spite of these factors, the Commission currently accepts that 'in many tax fields harmonisation is neither necessary nor desirable in view of the widely differing characteristics of Member States' tax systems and different national preferences' (European Commission 2001c: 9). In particular the Commission views taxes on personal income as a matter to be determined by the member states. Echoing many of the sentiments expressed by Tony Blair's Labour Government, the Commission today accepts that some degree of fair tax competition within the EU may contribute to lower tax pressures. Moreover, although the Commission does wish to see a limited approximation of member states' laws in the fields of environmental taxation, energy taxation and Value Added Tax (VAT), it accepts that the member states are likely to retain the veto in these areas for the foreseeable future.[9] For these reasons greater tax harmonisation resulting in lower welfare state expenditure at the national level cannot be seen as an inevitable consequence of EMU.

The economic policy mix

Today under EMU there is no single body to determine the optimal mix of monetary, fiscal and wage policies (Levitt and Lord 2000: 158). An effective policy mix is deemed essential to ensure all economic actors are contributing to the stability of the euro by pursuing complementary policy objectives. While monetary policy was centralised at the European level, economic policy remained at the national level becoming subject to the BEPGs and the much maligned Stability Pact (Dyson and Featherstone 1999: 788). As has been shown, the extent to which the current procedures have effectively coordinated the policies of the national fiscal authorities and the ECB's single monetary policy is questionable (Brunila *et al.* 2002: 18). At present, the relationship between the ECB and eurozone finance ministers remains on an uneasy basis as the ECB refuses to respond to demands from some member states for lower interest rates to stimulate growth, before it sees evidence of fiscal discipline and structural economic reform (FT.com, 1 February 2002, 20 May 2002).

It is clear that the ECB would prefer to react to one fiscal policy rather than 12 independent policies as at present. To this end the Commission President Romano Prodi has previously advocated the creation of a central fiscal institution. Any such centralisation would mark a significant stage in the process of political integration, given the important national functions fiscal policies fulfil. Yet as the current crisis with the performance of the Stability Pact has proved, attempts at reform have centred on measures to strengthen the existing procedures whereby national economic policies are coordinated at the European level.

As well as the measures designed to improve the interpretation and implementation of the SGP, these efforts have centred on developing a more constructive dialogue between the finance ministers and the ECB. To enable each actor to fully understand the consequences of their respective policies, attempts have been made to strengthen the Eurogroup – the informal grouping of finance ministers of participating member states (FT.com, 20 May 2002). Calls for the role of the Eurogroup to be strengthened have been made in the 2001 BEPGs and the Presidency conclusions of the Nice and Barcelona European Councils (Council of the European Union 2001a: 11, 2002b, 2002c: 4). As a result, the Eurogroup has started to extend the early exchange of information on an increased range of structural matters. Furthermore the Commission has also offered to involve itself more in the work of the Eurogroup, a proposal that has so far been resisted by the independently minded finance ministers.

Although the discussion has so far focused exclusively on the mix between monetary and fiscal policies, wage developments form a third important element of the macroeconomic policy mix. Under the single currency wages are far more comparable throughout the eurozone. However, a process of 'wage imitation' could jeopardise the stability of the euro if wage increases are not related to productivity gains, by forcing the ECB to raise the common interest rate (European Commission 2000e: 52–5). Furthermore, given the loss of other mechanisms for macroeconomic stabilisation, there is a greater need for flexibility within pay settlements to ensure they are responsive to broader economic trends. These factors have pushed the issue of wages onto the Community's agenda, despite the fact that from a formal treaty perspective, wages remain beyond the competence of the Community (Sciarra 1999: 167). In setting a common monetary policy, the ECB is faced with a highly organised, 'but extremely nationally fragmented system of wage setting' (Streeck 1998: 445). For this reason the EU is unlikely, in the foreseeable future, to be able to construct formal mechanisms to centralise wage setting at the European level. However, through the 'Cologne Process', efforts have been made to promote greater coordination among the relevant European-level actors (Council of the European Union 1999a) and create a new 'informal and open' tripartite European-level dialogue between the Social Partners, the Council and Commission, and representatives from the ECB (European Commission 2000d).

With the exception of the Cologne Process, efforts to ensure that wages contribute to an optimal policy mix have again centred on the coordination of national wage developments. This is a further function served by the soft-regulatory BEPGs. While the autonomy of the Social Partners is acknowledged, the member states are called upon to 'promote the right framework conditions for wage negotiations by [the] social partners' (European Commission 2002c: 12). The 2002 Guidelines require nominal wages to be consistent with price stability, and any increase in real wages not to exceed the growth of labour productivity. However, EMU is also contributing to a process of horizontal Europeanisation whereby national governments themselves are having to take a more active interest in wage developments as a result of European economic integration. As a result of EMU, national governments have lost a range of traditional tools for macroeconomic stabilisation. This has reconfigured the structure of power at the national level by increasing the importance of wage setting to the overall strength of the economy. Wages are now one of the few areas where governments can exert influence in respect of adjustment to economic shocks and maintenance of national competitiveness (Crouch 2000b: 224).

Together these EMU-induced factors have contributed to the (re-)emergence in some member states of national neo-corporatist arrangements to coordinate wage developments (Crouch 2000b: 209). During the 1990s EMU prompted the resurgence of national tripartite concertation in the form of social pacts in 11 member states (Streeck 1998: 444–5; European Commission 2000d). Although the rationale for, and content of, these pacts varied between countries, 'the common denominator' in all of them was strategies to enable governments and the Social Partners to mediate moderate wage settlements in a changed macro-economic environment (Crouch 2000b).

Should Britain join the single currency, these forces are unlikely to contribute to similar arrangements in the UK. Since a brief and unsuccessful flirtation with corporatist practices in the 1960s and 1970s, the combined effects of direct government action and the disorganised decentralisation of collective bargaining in Britain have destroyed 'virtually all mechanisms for coordinating bargaining at anything other than the most fragmented level' (Crouch 2000b: 222). The Social Partners are therefore not in a strong position to advance a process of coordination. Moreover, although the Labour Government has promoted a more consensual 'partnership approach' in industrial relations, this is extremely unlikely to extend to a major re-institutionalisation of the labour market necessary for the type of tripartite relationship that has evolved in other member states.

Overall, although EMU has provided a further impetus for integration in a range of ancillary policy areas, the fears of a forthcoming European superstate are clearly unfounded. In each of our cases, fiscal federalism, tax harmonisation and improving the policy mix, EMU did create pressures for greater centralisation. However, the distinctive interests and dynamics of the member states were more than a match for these tendencies. In these areas, the fears of EMU leading to a European political superstate that would undermine existing UK welfare state provisions and policies are clearly unfounded.

Conclusion

Overall, although the decision of 12 member states to proceed to full EMU has not exposed British monetary policy to any additional forces of vertical Europeanisation, the prior changes made by the Labour Government to the UK's monetary policy framework, such as Bank of England independence and price stability, do indicate a degree of horizontal Europeanisation. This does not imply the existence of any formal adaptational pressure exerted by the EU, but reflects a subtle process of cognitive convergence towards a dominant 'European' monetary policy framework that occurred throughout Europe during the 1980s and 1990s. By contrast, British budgetary policies *have* become subject to the soft-regulatory procedures of the Broad Economic Policy Guidelines, in particular the budget deficits and levels of debt constraints and emphasis on a state budget 'close to balance or surplus' by 2004. These objectives are broadly similar to the Government's current fiscal policy stance set in accordance with the 'golden rule' and 'sustainable investment rule'. Consequently, the European-level multilateral surveillance procedures have, to date, exerted little adaptational pressure on British economic policy.

If Britain joined the euro, there would be substantial institutional changes as the Bank of England would transfer national monetary policy control to the ECB. However, this transfer would be eased by the overall monetary policy similarities between the Bank of England and ECB. Furthermore, while Britain would lose the ability to devalue, current thinking is not supportive of this type of short-term stabilisation role for monetary policy. Concerns remain as to the effects a one-size-fits-all interest rate would have on the UK economy, the legitimacy of the ECB and the ability of the British Government to influence a fully established ECB. Nevertheless, as a large and important member state, the UK would probably obtain a high degree of flexibility in joining the euro, as demonstrated by the ability of the French and Germans to bend EMU rules. Moreover, although joining the euro would expose Britain to additional forces of vertical Europeanisation, the claims that EMU will inexorably lead to closer political union through the development of fiscal federalism, greater tax and economic policy harmonisation cannot be substantiated.

Finally, what does all of this imply for the UK welfare state? First, neither EMU nor the euro have radically altered the financial foundations or substantially harmonised the welfare states of the existing eurozone members. Like normal complex adaptive agents, the various member states have adjusted their budgetary and taxation policies to balance their particular demands and needs with the eurozone constraints. Unsurprisingly, larger countries have been able to stretch the EMU rules, while smaller countries have been more constrained. Nevertheless, as discussed at the start of this book, even the small countries have not seen a significant reduction in their welfare state expenditure. Second, since the EMU does not automatically lead to closer political union and further policy spillover, it is virtually impossible to predict the exact impact of the UK joining the euro on the welfare state. Overall, it would not be a radical change from the general UK economic policy mix, hence the normal healthy adaptive capacities of the UK welfare state would probably be capable of adjusting.

Notes

[1]   Protocol No. 25 (1992) on certain provisions relating to the United Kingdom of Great Britain and Northern Ireland (ex Protocol No. 11).

[2]   ESCB Statute Article 2.

[3]   Treaty Articles 2, 105.1.

[4]   Treaty Article 104 (ex Article 104c).

[5]   European Council Resolution, 17 June 1997 (97/C 235/01); Council Regulation (EC) 7 July 1997 No. 1466/97; Council Regulation (EC) 7 July 1997 No. 1467/97.

[6]   Council Regulation (EC) 7 July 1997 No. 1466/97.

[7]   The convergence programme that Britain is required to submit is similar in content to the stability programmes of the participating member states; however, it covers a broader range of variables including information on monetary policy objectives, notably with regard to inflation and exchange rates.

[8]   Treaty Article 116.4 (ex Article 109e.4).

[9]   Frustrated at Britain's negative response to calls for limited degree of tax harmonisation, Commission President Romano Prodi bemoaned 'tax is like sex, you cannot talk about that' (BBC News 2001).

Chapter 9

Conclusion: still a journey to an unknown destination

In this book we have tried to perform the difficult task of drawing together a macro-theoretical perspective with detailed case studies to make the fundamental arguments that the European Union (EU) and its impact on and relationship to UK social policy are emergent, complex and adaptive. Moreover, rather than being an irritation or indication of failure, the complex nature of the EU–UK social policy relationship is an important indicator of its evolving success and expansion. If this is true, how is it supported by the case studies and complexity theory? To answer that we must ask ourselves, what have we learned from the case studies and what can complexity theory tell us?

What have we learned from the case studies?

The impact of variable Europeanisation

As demonstrated by earlier works on EU social policy and confirmed by the most recent research,[1] the impact of Europeanisation in the UK is highly variable and complex and depends on the interwoven history of both EU and UK policy developments within a particular area. As our own case studies have shown, we have seen four different types of Europeanisation: coincidental, EU-led, partial and non-membership convergence.

In employment policy, the UK was not required to significantly alter its existing policy approach in order to conform to European requirements. This was generally due to the transformation of EU employment policy towards a more market-responsive, UK-oriented perspective. This coincidental convergence was not the result of a planned strategy, but evolved in response to the changing framework of global economic pressures on national economic strategies. In gender policy, the EU paralleled and occasionally led gender policy developments in the UK. This was due to the low level of gender policy advances in the UK, relative to other member states, and the unprecedented success of gender policy promoters at the EU level. In particular, it reflected the success of judicial strategies of EU gender policy promoters in entrenching gender policy in EU law and then using that law to evoke changes at the national level. In labour policy, there has been a partial Europeanisation of UK labour market policies. EU developments have helped to entrench a relative low floor of labour rights in the UK and encouraged the development of more consensual forms of labour–employer dialogue. This was due to pressures from the EU combining with internal political changes within the UK. Nevertheless, this has only been a partial transformation as many of the core voluntaristic elements of the UK labour market regime remain intact. Finally, non-membership in the European Monetary Union (EMU) has not meant that the UK has been able to pursue a radically independent economic strategy. In fact, if the UK were to join the EMU it would easily fit all of the core economic policy criteria. Interestingly, for primarily internal reasons the UK has pursued economic strategies that have led to a high degree of convergence with the EU.

Overall, we found a high degree of variation in both the adaptive pressures that the EU put on UK social policies and in the efforts with which UK actors implemented or resisted EU policies. This variation reflected both the multilevel nature of the relationship and the various political struggles continually occurring within different policy areas. For example, Labour Party support for particular polices often reflected both a desire to appear pro-EU at the European level, pro-workers' rights at a national level and split the Conservative Party at the party level. Often the Conservative Party opposed EU social policies primarily as a tactic for uniting their party. More fundamentally, there were core aspects and tendencies in the impact of Europeanisation on UK social policy, importance of EU legal initiatives, growing involvement in social issues, etc. However, the exact nature of that impact was distinctive in all of the areas we explored and we would expect a similar pattern to emerge in other social policy areas.

Emergence of new policy methods

As seen in the cases of gender and employment policy, the adoption of new and emergent policy methods is an ongoing part of the EU–UK policy process. For gender policy, we saw how a combination of national and EU level actors, frustrated by the limitations of traditional policy strategies, successfully embraced the mainstreaming tactic. As we saw, this tactic of promoting gender outside of its traditional policy arenas fitted in well with the capabilities of the EU level gender policy promoters, the structure of EU policy making and the shifting framework of European gender relations. Within the UK, gender mainstreaming was quickly adopted by gender policy promoters and resulted in a number of policy developments. However, it was also clear that mainstreaming cannot be generalised to all policy areas. On the one hand, it requires substantial political resources and a continuous multilevel effort. On the other hand, it is self-limiting. The more policy areas that are mainstreamed, the less any particular area benefits from the mainstreaming strategy. Hence, mainstreaming works best when only one group or policy area uses it. So far, gender policy has been that group. It remains to be seen how long this unique position can be maintained.

In employment policy, we saw the development of the 'open method of coordination' (OMC). In many ways, one could view this strategy as a response to failure. In most member states during the 1990s national level employment policies were struggling to deal with the continued challenges of unacceptably high levels of unemployment and long-term unemployed. At the same time, various EU level employment initiatives were discussed. However, with very different employment relations and policy regimes and the politically sensitive nature of this policy area, a large-scale, centrally driven EU employment policy was never a serious consideration. Given these limitations, a less traditional, more consensual and open process was one of the only ways forward. What emerged was a messy compromise of policy learning and political presentation. Most interestingly, the impact of the OMC seems to depend on the importance that national actors attach to it. As we saw in the British case, the OMC for employment policy was given a high profile within the Government, particularly since UK employment strategies fit so well with the Employment Guidelines. Obviously, it is open to question as to whether the UK Government would be so supportive of the OMC if its policies began to diverge from the guidelines. Nevertheless, the longer the OMC survives and becomes increasingly institutionalised within the EU policy process, the more one would expect its impact to increase.

Do institutions matter?

The simple answer is, of course they do. In each of our case studies, the interaction of the EU- and UK-level institutions was a major factor in the policy relationship. For example, in gender policy, the strength of EU and UK gender policy non-governmental organisations (NGOs) combined with the judicial strategy of these groups had a profound effect on the interrelated development of the EU–UK gender policy relationship. In labour policy, the traditional voluntaristic relationship between the main employer and employee organisations, the Confederation of British Industry (CBI) and the Trades Union Congress (TUC), greatly hampered the development of more cooperative and corporatistic strategies that EU labour policies like the Works Councils Directive implied. In employment, the dominance of the member state governments over the Employment Guidelines and OMC process means that both will remain at a very elite policy actor level. On the one hand, this will inhibit their impact on the wider array of employment policy actors. On the other hand, it may enable elite policy actors to actually learn from each other rather than focusing on purely political 'point-scoring' activities. Finally, the case of EMU raises a number of interesting issues. Joining the euro would obviously mean a significant transformation in the structure of monetary policy institutions. However, it would appear to have little impact on the economic fundamentals underlying the UK welfare state and social policy. Here governmental institutions have played less of a role than political parties and public opinion that, despite the economic arguments for or against, have significantly swayed the UK relationship towards EMU.

Overall, it is clear that institutions matter, they are central to any case study and their impact varies over time and policy areas. In all of our case studies they created 'pathways' that shaped policy outcomes. However, these pathways were neither deterministic nor universal to even our small number of policy areas.

Case studies as emergent complex adaptive processes

As demonstrated at the end of Chapters 5, 6 and 7, key elements of the EU–UK social policy relationship can be conceptualised and visualised as emergent complex adaptive processes. The elements of these processes can be divided into more orderly or disorderly aspects and an overall picture created of the complex nature of the policy relationship. There are several strengths and weaknesses of this type of conceptualisation. Its strengths include the ability to capture the multifaceted nature of the processes, the ubiquity of its application and capacity to separate the more predictable from the less predictable elements. Most observers of the EU–UK social policy process would have no difficulty in agreeing that the process is complex. It's obvious. It's common sense. The problem is that when one approaches this 'common sense' problem from a linear framework, one is forced to reduce it down to its component parts, trace out the cause and effect mechanisms and then try to prove that they exist. From a complexity framework, this reductionist attempt at causal determinism is doomed to failure and misleading. At best, we can talk in probabilities, but our ability to predict declines radically as we move along the range from orderly to disorderly phenomena. Visualising the elements of the EU–UK social policy relationship as complex phenomena keeps us from falling into this trap, and makes clear linkages to similarities with other types of complex phenomena.

Its weaknesses are the simplicity of the complexity divisions, the challenge of hidden complexity within and between each division and the problem of scale. In attempting to separate the various levels of complexity one is forced to radically simplify the complex interactions that are going on within and between the divisions. This is a constant limitation of any type of ideal-typical modelling and the cost of parsimony. The only qualification is that complexity theory constantly reinforces the point that one can never have complete deterministic knowledge of any emergent complex adaptive phenomena. Hence, there are always limits to knowledge and limits to representing reality. Finally, like aspects of fractal geometry, one can find complex emergent patterns at different levels or scales. For example, starting with key individual actors in UK social policy, the British Prime Minister or relevant ministers, their social policy decisions can easily be framed within a complexity framework. Moving upwards, one could then look at the larger dynamics of core groups in the social policy process, trade unions, NGOs, etc. Again, their actions could easily be placed into our order-to-disorder framework. This type of analysis could continue upwards until one was observing the complexity dynamics of global social policy developments. This cascade of complexity would seem to indicate that there is no end to the layers of complexity, and in a sense this would be true. However, just like the paradoxical nature of motion discussed by the ancient Greek, Zeno of Elea, who recognised that if you take the path of an arrow and then take half of it, then half of that and so on, you will still never return to your starting point. Nevertheless, in reality the arrow does hit its target and complexity phenomena do produce their outcome. Hence, the paradox of infinitesimals may challenge us theoretically, but not practically.

Next steps for case study research

Obviously we do not feel that we have exhausted the field of case study research on EU–UK social policy interaction. In fact, we have just barely scratched the surface. We have left unexplored whole areas of social policy including disability, education, health, youth, social security, etc. We see three key steps for the future of EU–UK policy research. First, in terms of EU–UK social policy interaction, more effort should be put into the continued comparative study of its sub-areas. A second step would be to compare the EU–UK social policy relationship with similar social policy areas in other member states. One might even explore the indirect effects of EU social policy on non-member states. A final step would be to begin to explore comparisons of the dynamics of the EU–UK social policy relationship with other policy fields both within the UK and other member states. None of these strategies are particularly radical or divergent from earlier research developments. The key point that a complexity framework would emphasise is that all of this research will not lead us to any sort of final knowledge of the EU–UK relationship. We must accept that our job is to illuminate the process as much as we can, recognise that we are part of the process, and see ourselves as facilitators to complex learning and decision-making activities of students, policy actors and informed voters. How they interpret our case studies and conclusions is a completely different layer of complexity!

What can complexity theory tell us?

Be aware of complexity

In one of the most forward-thinking, but unfortunately largely forgotten, works on European integration, Andrew Shonefield wrote that the EU was on a journey to an unknown destination (Shonefield 1972). Despite these early key insights most academics and a good part of the British public and media have desperately tried to fix the EU in one position or another ('a powermad super-state' or 'bloated bumbling bureaucracy'). These views reflect the entrenched nature of linear thinking in the UK rather than the complex reality of the EU. For the truth is, the EU is both and much more. Of course there are mistakes, confusion, misdirection and occasional corruption. No large complex social system exists without them. However, at its heart the EU is a complex adaptive system evolving in symbiosis with national, subnational and local-level member state complex adaptive systems in a context of an emergent global system. One can easily find examples of orderly, disorderly and complex phenomena within the EU and study those bits individually. However, one must always try to keep the larger complexity perspective in the frame.

Combine a broad fundamental framework with diversity

Most complex adaptive systems exist on what has been called 'the edge of chaos', the zone that combines basic fundamental rules with unpredictable combinations and random events to create a continual process of adaptation and emergence. Many of these adaptations fail. But, it is only by allowing the system to run through the possibilities that it becomes capable of responding to new situations and surviving. Unsurprisingly, in our chapters on key policy areas we found a substantial degree of healthy symbiotic variety. In employment policy, we saw a significant degree of coincidental convergence where the national and EU policy arenas mutually reinforced each other. In gender policy, the EU was actually leading the way in key areas. In labour market policy, European pressures affected a few areas, but did little to alter the fundamentally voluntaristic nature of the British system towards a more continental model. Finally, even the tremendous pressures of EMU seem very unlikely to radically alter the UK welfare state. This implies that the EU is not going to 'order' (save or destroy) the UK welfare state. What it has done is create a broad fundamental framework that impacts upon and interacts with different parts of the UK welfare state in distinctive ways. This diversity is not an indication of failure, as linear thinking would imply, but of strength. The exact nature of this diversity, the perfect point on the edge of chaos is unknowable and is an obvious frustration for linear thinkers. Nevertheless, it is the combination of a fundamental framework (the EU) with diverse adaptive responses from the multitude of national and subnational actors that makes complexity work.

Complexity and common sense

As the title of the book suggests, and as we have tried to show throughout, the interaction between the two levels is a far more complex process than has previously been acknowledged in academic work, and the aim must be to get away from simplistic linear models when explaining these processes. More importantly, complexity is the science of common sense. In our 70+ interviews with EU and UK policy actors we were constantly confronted with a sense of 'muddling through'. Most policy actors had a general framework, bounded by individual and institutional rules, norms and values, in which they were operating, though many professed never to think about it. However, most stressed that they never thought about the framework while pursuing their day-to-day decision making. Continually confronted with complicated and often contradictory detailed problems, opportunities and demands, they responded with a perpetual balancing act of sufficing, making-do or muddling-through behaviour. For them, the obvious point was that no framework or theory could possibly deal with or provide an answer to all of the micro-problems in their daily working lives. From a linear perspective, this common-sense behaviour is a fundamental problem or weakness. Central actors can and should create mechanisms (targets, quotas, criteria, etc) to minimise and if possible eliminate this muddling. The centre should be in control and can create appropriate outcomes from an orderly strategy. From a complexity perspective, the false belief in central control is much more dangerous than the daily muddling of decentralised actors. Real power lies in the millions of daily, incremental, small-scale and common-sense decisions that are taken every day by non-elite actors. Create a fundamental framework within which these actors can pursue their own disorderly pursuits, and a healthy complex system will emerge.

Decentralisation and the importance of local actors and interactions

This concept of local actor importance and autonomy runs counter to many of the deeply held traditions and beliefs of many British social policy academics and actors. In academic terms, the concept of the 'Westminster Model', whereby final decision making, control and responsibility rested in the hands of elite governmental actors, and the clear dominance of central governmental organisations in the development of social policy, sustained and justified the belief in central dominance and control (Ashford 1982). This framework has been criticised from a multitude of academic directions (Richards and Smith 2002). Nevertheless, as demonstrated by the targeting frenzy of the Blair government, it remains a core belief in the corridors of political power. However, as we have seen in our case studies the relationship between the UK and EU is influenced by much more than just dominant central actors. On the one hand, central actors are not really in control of the situation. They certainly have power and influence but, as we saw, the resulting policies can be a case of coincidental convergence, mutually reinforcing policies and/or resistant sub-actors and institutions. On the other hand, the decision making and interaction that does occur is not simply at a central government level (in this case defined as the Prime Minister, Cabinet members and elite civil servants), but also depends on a multitude of non-elite actors, such as lower level civil servants, political parties, social NGOs, local groups and so on. EU–UK social policy inter-action therefore is not a simple two-way street between the EU and government. From a complexity perspective, the ability of the EU to encourage the UK to escape from this centralising tendency is one of its fundamental bene-fits.

Re-conceptualising the EU–UK relationship: from 'awkward' to 'symbiotic' partner

Complexity does more than just challenge the centralising tendency in UK poli-tics, it also fundamentally reappraises the EU–UK relationship. Traditionally, the UK has been labelled an 'awkward' partner in its relationship to the EU, always dragging its feet in negotiations, opposing new European initiatives and seeing itself as more American than European (despite the fact that it is one of the fastest and most thorough implementers of EU legislation). For pro-Europeans in the UK this has been a significant embarrassment. For anti-Europeans, it has been something to be proud of. However, from a complexity perspective, the UK has a healthy symbiotic relationship with the EU. Like other member states, it is awkward in some areas, supportive in others, wins in some debates and loses in others, and embraces some changes and opposes others. By being awkward, the UK has been quite successful in shaping the EU social policy agenda in such a way as to make it suitable for itself. So, rather than labelling the UK an 'awkward' partner, one could actually say that, in the field of social policy at least, the UK has been very *successful*. On the one hand, it has resisted a variety of pressures from other actors to implement a more activist social policy agenda coming from 'Europe' while, on the other hand, actually managing to convince important actors within the EU that the way it manages the economy and the social costs of the free market is the 'right' way. This conclusion may be disappointing for pro-Europeans, but it is not a victory for anti-Europeans. In fact, the very success of the UK in defending its interests and objectives fundamentally undercuts the anti-European argument. In this sense, the EU–UK relationship is much more symbiotic than awkward.

The importance of adaptation, learning and innovation

Even more crippling for the Eurosceptic position are the fundamental benefits of EU–UK welfare state interaction, adaptation, learning and innovation. From a complexity perspective, there is nothing inherently final or supreme about the British welfare state. It is composed of a huge variety of complex adaptive actors and provides a number of socio-economic benefits, costs and opportunities for individual, group and societal development. Like other complex adaptive systems it needs to learn, adapt and innovate if it is going to successfully respond to the ever-changing needs and demands of its society. As seen in the case studies, the EU creates a stable framework for promoting interaction, adaptation, learning and innovation with the other main European welfare states and with itself. The exact outcome of this type of interaction is obviously very difficult to predict. Where UK labour, employment and gender policy will be in five years' time is virtually impossible to know in exact detail. However, one can predict with a high degree of certainty that a better policy will emerge if it is allowed to interact with other welfare state regimes.

Complexity and the welfare state

More broadly, complexity is not wedded to any particular type of advanced welfare state. The American, Dutch, German, Norwegian, Swiss, etc all have distinctive attributes that have emerged through lengthy and unique historical processes. One can easily make a variety of arguments for or against particular aspects of any of these systems, but to say which one is the best and then try to shift it into your own system and believe that the same outcomes will be produced is both foolish and dangerous. What complexity does imply is that the society that is the most complex, with the largest amount of interaction, adaptation, learning and innovation going on within it, will be the most likely to successfully respond to the inevitable changes that will confront it in the future. There is no final welfare state, nor is a given type of welfare state an end in itself. What one needs to do is avoid the belief that certain institutions and policies are fixed and final, as 'third way' thinking implies, regarding the future of society as an inevitable compromise between states and markets. Complexity argues that there is no known endpoint to work towards. If history teaches us anything, it is that there are always different paths to follow and different ways to go down those paths. In short, there is not only a third way, but a fourth, fifth, sixth, etc way as well. The key for policy actors is to put in place fundamental structures that encourage the maximum amount of decentralised interaction, adaptation, innovation and learning within their given societies. These abilities will enable the societies to prosper whatever 'way' they eventually choose.

Complexity, the EU and European civil society

Obviously, complexity does not just apply to the member state level. In general, due to its relative weakness the EU is unable to overly order the member states. But this doesn't stop it from trying. As at the member state level, the EU should avoid attempting to overly order member state welfare states and civil societies, and do more to encourage interaction between the various member state systems. The EU, due to its multilevel and decentralised structure, tends to pursue complexity maximising strategies that often involve civil society. Thus, there is a general institutional affinity between the EU and civil society. As most observers will note, European civil society varies significantly between nation-states. Moreover, within each national system there is a huge variety of civil society organisational forms. In the past decade the EU did much to try and support the creation of some form of European civil society. Basically, this is a good idea, but the EU should avoid trying to pick or promote a given type of organisational form for civil society actors. An example of attempts to do this can be found in the debates over the funding of EU social and civil groups (Geyer 2001). Fundamentally, the EU will have no way of knowing whether a given form is correct for all situations. The attempt to impose such a form would lead to a significant political backlash. And, if successfully imposed, it would significantly weaken the complexity of the system.

Instead, the EU should promote symbiotic competition between national-level civil society systems. Most civil society systems in the member states are dynamic learning systems within ordered environments. However, if these systems are to increase their complexity and hence learning, adaptation and innovation skills, encouraging interaction between the national systems is an obvious step. Again, this should not be imposed from above through a strategy of harmonisation, but through an opening up of the civil society activities between member states. Examples could include the ability of civil society organisations to organise and/or offer services in other member states (health sector and pension services are obvious possibilities). In essence, this implies a 'mutual recognition' of civil society systems in the various member states and the rights of individuals and societies to access and take advantage of different systems. The job of the EU would be to open up the 'nationalised' civil society systems and encourage interaction, adaptation and learning.

Clearly, not only should the EU promote interaction between the nation-alised civil society systems, but it should also promote the creation of a European civil society. In many ways, one could see this as a similar project to the creation of a European free market. National systems would continue, but would be encouraged to learn and innovate through interaction with other national systems and a European system. European civil society could be promoted through regulatory and legislative proposals and through basic funding, steps that the EU is already taking. Like the promotion and protection of infant industries, European civil society would require a degree of support and protection, particularly in its early stages. An example of this type of support already exists in the EU's promotion of the social and civil dialogue and funding of social and civil European actors. Arguably, if the EU wants to increasingly promote a European civil society, it would need to substantially increase its political and financial support for that system.

Lastly, of the three main systems, the civil society is the weakest at the European level. Market interaction and integration have accelerated radically since the 1970s. Similarly, state interaction within the EU institutions and between the member states has increased dramatically since the 1980s. On the other hand, European civil society is in its emerging stages. There is little intra-member state system interaction and uneven development at the European level. If the EU were to significantly promote a European civil society, European market and state actors would be likely to feel threatened and oppose it. In response to this, the EU should do what it can to protect the European civil society from these fundamental threats. Basically, the more the EU is capable of providing a stable framework for the expansion of European civil society activities, the more social and civil actors will be able to interact, learn and take risks within their environment. Consequently, the more the European civil society will create a symbiotic competition with the other sectors that will strengthen all three. Fundamentally, the EU must argue that promoting civil society is a way of promoting greater complexity within all of the sectors and thus greater adaptation, learning and innovation within the European society as a whole.

Final point

In sum, complexity is not a magic formula for solving the detailed problems of social policy actors at the subnational, national or European level. What it does do is provide a scientific framework for understanding why the millions of daily micro-decisions taken by non-elite actors, based on local muddling through, actually result in reasonable global outcomes. Elite actors can and should try to nudge this activity in what they think is the right direction. However, they must constantly realise that they do not possess final knowledge of the system, and that they can achieve much more by providing a fundamental framework for the local actors and allowing local actors to find their own complex solutions. With complexity, elites may actually be able to achieve more by doing less.

Note

[1] Ian Bache at the University of Sheffield has been directing a major ESRC/UACES research project into 'The Europeanization of British politics and policy-making'. For more information *see*: www.shef.ac.uk/ebpp/.

References

Abbott D (2000) The case against the Maastricht model of central bank independence. In: M Baimbridge, B Burkitt and P Whyman (eds) *The Impact of the Euro. Debating Britain's future*. Macmillan, Basingstoke. 220–36.

Adler E (1997) Seizing the middle ground: constructivism in World politics. *European Journal of International Relations* 3: 319–63.

Adnett N and Hardy S (2001) Reviewing the Working Time Directive: rationale, implementation and case law. *Industrial Relations Journal*. 32: 114–25.

Allen P (2001) What is Complexity Science? *Emergence*. 3: 1.

Allison G (1971) *The Essence of Decision: explaining the Cuban Missile Crisis*. Little Brown, Boston.

Alter KJ and Vargas J (2000) Explaining variation in the use of litigation strategies. European community law and British gender equality policy. *Comparative Political Studies*. 33: 452–82.

Ardy B and Begg I (2001) *The European Employment Strategy: policy integration by the back door*. Paper prepared for the ECSA 7th Biennial Conference, Madison, Wisconsin, 31 May–2 June 2001. www.sbu.ac.uk/euroinst/401.pdf (accessed 8 September 2004).

Arestis P and Sawyer M (2000) The deflationary consequences of the single currency. In: M Baimbridge, B Burkitt and P Whyman *et al*. (eds) *The Impact of the Euro. Debating Britain's future*. Basingstoke: Macmillan. 100–12.

Armstrong K and Shaw J (1998) Integrating law: an introduction. *Journal of Common Market Studies*. 36: 2.

Ashley R (1986) The poverty of neorealism. In: R Keohane (ed.) *Neorealism and its Critics*. Columbia University Press, New York. 255–300.

Axelrod R (1997) *The Complexity of Cooperation*. Princeton University Press, Princeton, NJ.

Axelrod R and Cohen MD (2000) *Harnessing Complexity: organizational implications of a scientific frontier*. The Free Press, New York.

Axtmann R (ed.) (1998) *Globalization and Europe: theoretical and empirical investigations*. Pinter, London.

Bachtler J and Turock I (eds) (1997) *The Coherence of EU Regional Policy: contrasting perspectives on the structural funds*. Regional Policy and Development Series 17, Regional Studies Association, Jessica Kingsley Publishers, London.

Bagilhole B (1997) *Equal Opportunities and Social Policy*: issues of gender, race and disability. Addison Wesley Longman, Harlow.

Bainbridge T (1998) *The Penguin Companion To European Union*. Penguin Books, London.

Barnard C (1994) A European litigation strategy: the case of the Equal Opportunities Commission. In: J Shaw and G More (eds) *New Legal Dynamics of the European Union*. Oxford University Press, Oxford. 254–72.

Barnard C (2000a) *EC Employment Law* (2e). Oxford University Press, Oxford.

Barnard C (2000b) The Working Time Regulations 1999. *Industrial Law Journal*. 29: 167–75.

Barnett W, Geweke J and Shell K (eds) (1989) *Economic Complexity: chaos, sunspots, bubbles and non-linearity*. Cambridge University Press, Cambridge.

Barrow J, Davies P and Harper C (eds) (2004) *Science and Ultimate Reality: quantum theory, cosmology and complexity*. Cambridge University Press, Cambridge.

Bar-Yam Y (1997) *Dynamics of Complex Systems*. Perseus Press, Reading.

BBC News (2001) *Non-Euro Britain Losing Influence*. 15 February. www.news. bbc.co.uk/1/hi/uk_politics/1171374.stm (accessed 23 March 2005).

Beck U (1992) *The Risk Society: towards a new modernity*. Polity Press, Cambridge.

Begg I and Mayes D (1993) Cohesion, convergence and economic and monetary union in Europe. *Regional Studies.* **27**: 149–65.

Benton T (1999) Radical politics – neither left nor right. In: M O'Brien, S Penna and C Hay (eds) *Theorising Modernity: reflexivity, environment and identity in Giddens' social theory*. Longman, London. 80–102.

Bercusson B (1996) *European Labour Law*. Butterworths, London.

Beveridge F, Nott S and Stephen K (2000a) Setting the scene: the why, what and how of promoting equality between the sexes. In: F Beveridge, S Nott and K Stephen (eds) *Making Women Count: integrating gender into law and policy-making*. Ashgate Dartmouth, Aldershot. 1–23.

Beveridge F, Nott S and Stephen K (2000b) Making women count in the United Kingdom. In: F Beveridge, S Nott and K Stephen (eds) *Making Women Count: integrating gender into law and policy-making*. Ashgate Dartmouth, Aldershot. 163–90.

Beveridge FS, Nott S and Stephen K (2000c) Mainstreaming and the engendering of policy-making: a means to an end? *Journal of European Public Policy.* **7**(3) **Special Issue**: 385–405.

Bevir M (1999) *The Logic of the History of Ideas*. Cambridge University Press, Cambridge.

Bhaskar R (1986) *Scientific Realism and Human Emancipation*. Verso, London.

Biagi M (1998) The implementation of the Amsterdam Treaty with regard to employment: coordination or convergence. *International Journal of Comparative Labour Law and Industrial Relations.* **14**: 325–36.

Biagi M (2001) Quality in community industrial relations: an institutional viewpoint. *International Journal of Comparative Labour Law and Industrial Relations.* **17**: 385–94.

Blanpain R and Engels C (1998) *European Labour Law*. Kluwer Law International, The Hague.

Bomberg E and Peterson J (2000) *Policy Transfer and Europeanization*. Europeanisation Online Papers, Queen's University Belfast, 2/2000 www.qub.ac.uk (accessed 1 March 2005).

Bonoli G, George V and Taylor-Gooby P (2000) *European Welfare Futures: towards a theory of retrenchment*. Polity Press, Cambridge.

Boyer R and Drache D (1996) *States Against Markets: the limits of globalization*. Routledge, London.

Brewster C and Teague P (1989) *European Community Social Policy: its impact on the UK*. Institute for Personnel Management, London.

Brittan L (2000) *A Diet Of Brussels: the changing face of Europe*. Little, Brown and Company, London.

Brittan S (1977) The economic tension of British democracy. In: R Emmett Tyrrell Jr. (ed.) *The Future That Doesn't Work: Social Democracy's failures in Britain*. Doubleday, New York. 126–43.

Broad R and Preston V (eds) (2001) *Moored to the Continent? Britain and European integration*. Institute of Historical Research, London.

Brunila A, Buti M and Franco D (eds) (2002) *The Stability and Growth Pact: the architecture of fiscal policy in EMU*. Palgrave Macmillan Publishers, Basingstoke.

Brunn N (2001) The European Employment Strategy and the 'Acquis Communitaire' of labour law. *International Journal of Comparative Labour Law and Industrial Relations*. **14**: 325–36.

Burrows N and Mair J (1996) *European Social Law*. John Wiley Sons Ltd, Chichester.

Buti M, Eijffinger S and Franco D (2003) Revisiting the Stability and Growth Pact: grand design or internal adjustment. *European Economy Economic Papers*, No. 180, January 2003. European Commission, Brussels. www.europa.eu.int/comm./economy_finance/publications/economic_papers/economic-papers180_en.htm

Byrne D (1998) *Complexity Theory and the Social Sciences*. Routledge, London.

Cabinet Office website. www.cabinet-office.gov.uk

Capra F (1991) *The Tao of Physics*. Shambhala Publications, Boston.

Capra F (1996) *The Web of Life*. HarperCollins, New York.

Carley M and Hall M (2000) The implementation of the European Works Councils Directive. *Industrial Law Journal*. **29(2)**: 103–23.

CBI (2001a) *CBI Praises Government for Negotiating 'Least Damaging' Deal on Consultation Law*. News Release 17 December 2001. www.cbi.org/ndbs/press/nsf/

CBI (Confederation of British Industry) (2001b) *European Proposals on national-level information and consultation*. www.cbi.org

CBI (2003) *Maintaining a Dynamic Labour Market: The Working Time Directive and the individual opt-out*. Confederation of British Industries, London. www.cbi.org.uk/ndbs/press.nsf/0353c1f07c6ca12a8025671c00381cc7?25d7307dd360bf880256d4f002e09d0/$FILE/Working+Time+Report.pdf

Cerny PG (1990) *The Changing Architecture of Politics*. Sage, London.

Checkel J (1998) The constructivist turn in international relations theory. *World Politics*. **50**: 324–48.

Checkel J (1999) Social construction and integration. *Journal of European Public Policy*. **6**: 545–60.

Christiansen T, Jørgensen KE and Wiener A (2001) *The Social Construction of Europe*. Sage, London.

Chryssochoou D (2001) *Theorizing European Integration*. Sage, London.

Cilliers P (1998) *Complexity and Postmodernism: understanding complex systems*. Routledge, London.

Cioffi-Revilla C (1998) *Politics and Uncertainty*. Cambridge University Press, Cambridge.

Clarke J, Gewirtz S and McLaughlin E (eds) (2000) *New Managerialism, New Welfare?* Sage, London.

Cochrane A, Clarke J and Gerwirtz S (eds) (2001) *Comparing Welfare States*. Sage, London.

Colaianni T (1996) *European Works Councils: a legal and practical guide*. Sweet Maxwell, London.

Council of Europe (1998) *Gender Mainstreaming: conceptual framework, methodology and presentation of good practices*. Strasbourg (EG-S-MS (98) 2).

Council of the European Communities (1982) *Council Resolution 82/C 186/03 on the Promotion of Equal Opportunities for Women* (OJ 1982 C186).

Council of the European Communities (1990) *Council Recommendation 91/131 on the Protection of the Dignity of Women and Men at Work* (OJ 1990 C157).

Council of the European Union (1997a) *Resolution of the European Council on the Stability and Growth Pact; Amsterdam, 17 June 1997* (97/C 236/01) (OJC, 236, 2.8.1997).

Council of the European Union (1997b) *Council Regulation of 7 July 1997 on the Strengthening of the Surveillance of Budgetary Positions and the Surveillance and Coordination of Economic Policies.* No. 1466/97 (OJL, 209, 2.8.1997).

Council of the European Union (1997c) *Council Regulation of 7 July 1997 on Speeding up and Clarifying the Implementation of the Excessive Deficit Procedure.* No. 1467/97 (OJL, 209, 2.8.1997).

Council of the European Union (1998) *Presidency Conclusions – Cardiff European Council 15 and 16 June 1998.*

Council of the European Union (1999a) *Council Directive 99/70/EC of 28 June 1999 concerning the Framework Agreement on Fixed-term Work concluded by UNICE, CEEP and the ETUC.*

Council of the European Union (1999b) Council Regulation (EC) No. 1260/1999 of 21 June 1999 laying down general provisions on the Structural Funds (OJ 1999 L161/1).

Council of the European Union (1999c) *Council Resolution of 22 February 1999 on the 1999 Employment Guidelines* (OJ 1999 C69/02).

Council of the European Union (2000) *Presidency Conclusions – Lisbon European Council 23 and 24 March 2000.*

Council of the European Union (2001a) *Council Recommendation of 15 June 2001 on the Broad Economic Guidelines of the Economic Policies of the Member States and the Community* (9326/01).

Council of the European Union (2001b) *Council Recommendation of 19 January 2001 on the implementation of Member States' employment policies.* (2001/64/EC) (OJL, 22 24.1.2001).

Council of the European Union (2001c) *Council Decision of 19 January 2001 on Guidelines for Member States' employment policies for the year 2001.* (2001/63/EC) (OJL, 22, 24.1.2001).

Council of the European Union (2002a) *Council Directive 2002/73/EC amending Council Directive 76/207/EEC on the Implementation of the Principle of Equal Treatment for Men and Women as Regards Access to Employment, Vocational Training and Promotion and Working Conditions.*

Council of the European Union (2002b) *Council Decision of 18 February 2002 on Guidelines for Member States' Employment Policies for the Year 2002.* (2002/177/EC) (OJL, 60, 1.3.2002).

Council of the European Union (2002c) *Council Recommendation of 18 February 2002 on the Implementation of Member States' Employment Policies.* (2002/178/EC) OJL, 60, 1.3.2002.

Council of the European Union (2003) *Council Opinion of 18 February 2003 on the Updated Convergence Programme of the United Kingdom 2001/02 to 2007/08* (OJC, 051, 5.3.2003).

Coveney P and Highfield R (1992) *The Arrow of Time: a voyage through science to solve time's greatest mystery.* Fawcett Books, London.

Coveney P and Highfield R (1995) *Frontiers of Complexity: the search for order in a chaotic world.* Faber and Faber, London.

Cowles MG, Caporaso J and Risse T (eds) (2001) *Transforming Europe: Europeanization and domestic change.* Cornell University Press, Ithaca.

Craig P and de Burca G (1995) *EC Law Text, Cases and Materials.* Oxford University Press, Oxford.

Craig P and Harlow C (eds) (1998) *The European Law-Making Process.* Kluwer, Deventer.

Cram L (1997) *Policy-Making in the European Union: conceptual lenses and the integration process.* Routledge, London.

Crawford M (1996) *One Money for Europe*: *the economics and politics of EMU.* Macmillan Press Ltd, Basingstoke.

Crawley C and Slowey J (1995) *Women and Europe, 1985–1995.* Birmingham Voluntary Service Council, Birmingham.

Cressey P (1993) Employee participation. In: M Gold (ed.) *The Social Dimension. Employment policy in the European Community.* Macmillan, London. 85–104.

Crompton R (1997) *Women and Work in Modern Britain.* Oxford University Press, Oxford.

Crouch C (2000a) Introduction: the political and institutional deficits of European Monetary Union. In: C Crouch (ed.) *After The Euro. Shaping institutions for governance in the wake of European Monetary Union.* Oxford University Press, Oxford. 1–23.

Crouch C (2000b) National wage determination and European Monetary Union. In: C Crouch (ed.) *After The Euro. Shaping institutions for governance in the wake of European Monetary Union.* Oxford University Press, Oxford. 203–26.

Currie D (1999) *The Pros and Cons of EMU,* An updated summary of a report published by the Economist Intelligence Unit in February 1997. www. hm-treasury.gov.uk/pub/html/docs/emupc/main.html (accessed 7 September 2004).

Dahrendorf R (1999) Whatever happened to liberty? *New Statesman.* **6 September**: 25–7.

Day R and Samuelson P (1994) *Complex Economic Dynamics.* The MIT Press, Boston.

de la Porte C (2002) Is the open method of coordination appropriate for organising activities at European level in sensitive areas? *European Law Journal.* **8**: 38–58.

de la Porte C, Pochet P and Room G (2001) Social bench marking, policy making and new governance in the EU. *Journal of European Social Policy.* 11: 291–307.

de Schoutheete P (2001) The misunderstood euro. *FT.com Financial Times* 29 August 2001. www.news.ft.com/ft/ (accessed 7 September 2004).

Degryse C and Pochet P (2001) The European employment strategy after Lisbon: from strategy to intention? In: C Degryse and P Pochet (eds) *Social Policy in the European Union 2000.* European Trade Union Institute, Brussels.

Delanty G (1997) *Social Science: beyond constructivism and realism.* Open University Press, Buckingham.

Department for Education and Employment (DfEE) (1998) *United Kingdom Employment Action Plan 1998.* DfEE, London.

DfEE (1999) *United Kingdom Employment Action Plan 1999.* www.dwp.gov. uk/eap/index.htm

DfEE (2000) *United Kingdom Employment Action Plan 2000.* www.dwp.gov. uk/eap/index.htm

DfEE (2001) *United Kingdom Employment Action Plan 2001.* www.dwp.gov.uk/ publications/dwp/2001/eactpln/enap2k1.pdf (accessed 2 March 2005).

DfEE, Department of Social Security and HM Treasury (2001) *Towards Full Employment in a Modern Society.* www.dwp.gov.uk/fullemployment/

Diez T (1999) Speaking 'Europe': the politics of integration discourse. *Journal of European Public Policy.* **6**: 598–613.

Dolowitz D and Marsh D (1996) Who learns what from whom: a review of the policy transfer literature. *Political Studies.* **44**: 343–57.

Dreamer D and Fleischaker G (1992) *Origins of Life: central concepts.* Jones and Bartlett Publishers, Boston.

Driver S and Martell L (2000) Left, Right and the Third Way. *Policy and Politics.* **28**: 2, 147–61.

DSS (1998) *A New Contract on Welfare.* HMSO, London.

DSS (1999) *Opportunity for All: tackling poverty and social exclusion.* HMSO, London.

DTI (1998) *Fairness At Work* (White Paper). www.dti.gov.uk/er/fairness/ index.htm (accessed 2 March 2005).

DTI (1999a) *Employees' Information and Consultation Rights on Collective Redundancies and Transfers of Undertakings. A short guide to the new requirements.* URN 99/1036. www.dti.gov.uk/er/consultation/redundancy.htm (accessed 2 March 2005).

DTI (1999b) *Transnational Information and Consultation of Employees Regulations 1999. Guidance Note.* www.dti.gov.uk/er/consultation/ewcover2.htm (accessed 2 March 2005).

DTI (1999c) *Outcome of the Public Consultation of the Implementation of the European Works Councils Directive.* www.dti.gov.uk/er/outcome2.pdf (accessed 2 March 2005).

DTI (1999d) *Implementation in the UK of the European Works Councils Directive.* URN 99/926.

DTI (2000) *Work Parents: competitiveness and choice* (Green Paper). www.dti.gov. uk/er/g_paper/index.htm (accessed 2 March 2005).

DTI (2002a) *Paternity – Leave and Pay. A basic summary.* www.dti.gov.uk/er/individual/paternity-p1514.htm

DTI (2002b) *Amendments to the Part-time Workers (Prevention of Less Favourable Treatment) Regulations 2000.* www.dti.gov.uk/er/fixed/ptime.htm (accessed 2 March 2005).

DTI European Structural Funds website: www.dti.gov.uk/europe/ structural.html (accessed 2 March 2005).

Duff A (1997) *The Treaty of Amsterdam: text and commentary.* Federal Trust, London.

DWP (2001) *United Kingdom National Action Plan on Social Inclusion 2001–2003.* www.dss.gov.uk/publications.dss/2001/Uknapsi/uknap2001_03.pdf

DWP (2002) *United Kingdom Employment Action Plan 2002.* www.hm-treasury. gov.uk/mediastore/otherfiles/emp_plan02.pdf (accessed 2 March 2005).

Dyson K (2000) EMU as Europeanisation: convergence, diversity and contingency. *Journal of Common Market Studies.* **38**: 645–66.

Dyson K and Featherstone K (1999) *The Road to Maastricht: negotiating Economic and Monetary Union.* Oxford University Press, Oxford.

Eagleton T (1996) *The Illusion of Postmodernism.* Blackwell Publishers, Oxford.

Economist Economic Focus (1998) Can one size fit all? *Economist*. 28 March.

ECOTEC Research and Consulting Limited (2002) *UK Contribution to the Evaluation of the European Employment Strategy*. ECOTEC Research and Consulting Limited, London.

Edwards P (1995) *Industrial Relations. Theory and practice in Britain*. Blackwell Publishers, Oxford.

Edwards P, Hall M, Hyman R *et al.* (1992) Great Britain: still muddling through. In R Hyman and A Ferner (eds) *Industrial Relations in the New Europe*. Blackwell, Oxford. 1–68.

Eichengreen B (2000) Saving Europe's automatic stabilisers. In: M Baimbridge, B Burkitt and P Whyman (eds) *The Impact of the Euro. Debating Britain's future*. Macmillan, Basingstoke.

EIRO (European Industrial Relations Observatory) (1997a, April) *The Industrial Relations Consequences of the 'New' Labour Government*. www.eiro.eurofound.ie.1997/04/Feature/UK9704125F.html

EIRO (1997b, August) *Employee Representation: new challenges from Europe*. www.eiro.eurofound.ie/1997/08/features/uk9708152.html

EIRO (1998, October) *New Working Time Regulations Take Effect*. www.eiro. eurofound.ie.1998/10/Feature/UK9810154F.html

EIRO (1999a, August) *Government Unveils Proposals for Statutory Parental Leave*. www.eiro.eurofound.ie/1999/08/inbrief/uk9901123N.html (accessed 2 March 2005).

EIRO (1999b, April) *The UK's First National Minimum Wage*. www. eiro.eurofound.ie/1999/04/Feature/UK9904196F.html (accessed 2 March 2005).

EIRO (1999c, March) *TUC Poll Highlights Case for Parental Leave to be Paid. European Foundation for the Improvement of Living and Working Conditions*.

EIRO (1999d, February) *Non-union Forms of Employee Representation*. www.eiro.eurofound.ie/1999/02/Features/uk9901181.html (accessed 2 March 2005).

EIRO (1999e, July) *New Directive Set to Improve Rights of Fixed-term Contract Workers*. www.eiro.eurofound.ie/1999/07/Feature/EU9907181F.html (accessed 2 March 2005).

EIRO (1999f, July) *Government Proposes Changes to Working Time Regulations*. www.eiro.eurofound.ie/1999/07/InBrief/uk9907117

EIRO (1999g, March) *Trade Union Recognition and the Employment Relations Bill*. www.eurofound.ie/1999/03/Features/uk9903189

EIRO (1999h, May) *Labour's 'Family-friendly' Employment Agenda*. www.eiro.eurofound.eu.int/1999/05/feature/uk9905103f.html (accessed 23 March 2005).

EIRO (2000a, December) *2000 Annual Review for the UK*. www.eiro.eurofound. ie./2000/12/features/UK0012109

EIRO (2000b, January) *The Impact of the 1998 Working Time Regulations*. www.eiro.eurofound.ie/2000/01/Features/uk0001150

EIRO (2000c, May) *Regulations introduce New Rights for Part-Time Workers*. www.eiro.eurofound.ie.2000/05/Features/uk0005175F.html

EIRO (2000d, July) *Statutory Trade Union Recognition Procedure Comes into Force*. www.eiro.eurofound.ie/2000/07/Feature/UK0007183F.html (accessed 2 March 2005)

EIRO (2001a, December) *Parents to Have Legal Right to Request Flexible Working.* www.eiro.eurofound.ie.2001/12/InBrief/UK0112105N.html

EIRO (2001b, August) *UK Implementation of the Fixed-Term Work Directive Delayed.* www.eiro.eurofound.ie/2001/08InBriefUK0108141N.html

EIRO (2001c, July) *UK Holiday Rule Unlawful says ECJ.* www.217.141.24.196/2001/01/inbrief/UK0107138N.html

EIRO (2001d, March) *Advocate-General finds against UK in ECJ Working Time Case.* www.eiro.eurofound.ie/2001/03/InBrief/UK0103118N.html (accessed 2 March 2005).

EIRO (2001e, October) *Government Announces Changes to Working Time Regulations.* www.217.141.24.196/2001/10/InBrief/UK0110105N.html

EIRO (2001f, April) *EOC Urges New Action on Equal Pay.* www.eiro.eurofound.ie.2001/04feature/UK0104126F.html (accessed 23 March 2005).

EIRO (2001g, February) *Government Calls for a Better Work-Life Balance.* www.eiro.eurofound.ie/2001/02/Feature/UK0102115F.html

EIRO (2002a, April) *Final Approval Given to Consultation Directive.* www.eiro.eurofound.ie.2001/02/Feature/UK0102115F.html (accessed 23 March 2005).

EIRO (2002b, February) *Unions Challenge the UK's Long Hours Culture.* www.217.141.24.196/2002/01/Feature/UK0101102F.html

EIRO (2002c, January) *UK Reaction to Agreement on EU Employee Consultation Directive.* www.217.141.24.196/print/2002/01/inbrief/UK0201116N.html

EIRO (2002d, June) *European Company Statute in Focus.* www.eiro.eurofound.ie/2002/06/Feature/EU0206202F.html (accessed 2 March 2005).

EIRO (2002e, October) *Employment Act 2002 Outlined.* www.eiro.eurofound.ie.2002/10/Feature/UK0210103F.html

EIRR (European Industrial Relations Review) (1996) New consultation rights for employee representatives. *EIRR.* **264**: 28–31.

EIS (European Information Service) (2000) **209.** www.eisnet.eis.be

Ellison N and Pierson C (2003) (eds) *New Developments in British Social Policy.* Palgrave, London.

EOC (Equal Opportunities Commission) (2001) *25 Legal Cases.* www.eoc.org.uk.cseng/legislation/25 legal cases.asp

EOC (2002a) *What does the Equal Pay Act say?* www.eoc.org.uk/cseng/legislation/the_sex_discrimination_act_an_overview.asp (accessed 2 March 2005).

EOC (2002b) *What does the Sex Discrimination Act say?* www.eoc.org.uk/cseng/legislation/the_sex_discrimination_act_an_overview.asp (accessed 2 March 2005).

EOC (2002c) *About the EOC.* www.eoc.org.uk/cseng/abouteoc/abouteoc.asp (accessed 2 March 2005).

EOC (2002d) *Work–Life Balance.* www.eoc.org.uk/cseng.policyandcampaings/work-life_balance.asp

Esping-Andersen G (1985) *Politics Against Markets: The Social Democratic road to power.* Princeton University Press, Princeton, NJ.

Esping-Andersen G (1996) *Welfare States in Transition.* Sage, London.

European Commission (1990) *Community Charter of the Fundamental Social Rights of Workers.* Office for Official Publications of the European Communities, Luxembourg.

European Commission (1993a) White Paper, *Growth Competitiveness and Employment: the challenges and ways forward into the 21st century*. Bull E, Supp C, 6/93. Office for the Official Publications of the European Communities, Luxembourg.

European Commission (1993b) Green Paper, *European Social Policy: options for the Union*. COM(93) 551 final of 17.11.93. Office for the Official Publications of the European Communities, Luxembourg.

European Commission (1994) White Paper, *European Social Policy: a way forward for the Union*. COM(94) 333 final/2 of 27.7.94. Office for the Official Publications of the European Communities, Luxembourg.

European Commission (1996) *Communication from the Commission: incorporating equal opportunities for women and men into all Community policies and activities*. Brussels, 21.2.1996 COM(96) 67 final. Office for the Official Publications of the European Communities, Luxembourg.

European Commission (1998) *Social Action Programme 1998–2000*. Office for Official Publications of the European Communities, Luxembourg.

European Commission (1999a) *Report from the Commission on the Implementation of the Council Directive 92/85/EEC of 19 October 1992 on the Introduction of Measures to Encourage Improvements in the Health and Safety at Work of Pregnant Workers and Workers who have Recently Given Birth or who are Breastfeeding.* Brussels, 15.03.1999 COM(1999) 100 final. Office for the Official Publications of the European Communities, Luxembourg.

European Commission (1999b) *The European Employment Strategy: investing in people, investing in more and better jobs*. Office for the Official Publications of the European Communities, Luxembourg.

European Commission (2000a) *Communication from the Commission to the Council, the European Parliament, the Economic and Social Committee and the Committee of the Regions. Towards a Community framework strategy on gender equality*. Brussels, 7.6.2000 COM(2000) 335 final. Office for the Official Publications of the European Communities, Luxembourg.

European Commission (2000b) *The Commission and Non-Governmental Organisations: building a stronger partnership*. EC, Brussels.

European Commission (2000c) *European Employment and Social Policy: a policy for people*. EC, Brussels.

European Commission (2000d) *Industrial Relations in Europe – 2000 Report*. Brussels, 06.03.2000 COM(2000) 113 final. Office for the Official Publications of the European Communities, Luxembourg.

European Commission (2000e) *Joint Employment Report 2000*. Brussels, 6.9.2000 COM(2000) 551 final. Office for the Official Publications of the European Communities, Luxembourg.

European Commission (2001a) *EU employment and social policy, 1999–2001, Jobs, Cohesion, Productivity.* Office for the Official Publications of the European Communities, Luxembourg.

European Commission (2001b) *Joint Employment Report 2001*. Brussels, 12.9.2001 COM(2001) 438 final. Office for the Official Publications of the European Communities, Luxembourg.

European Commission (2001c) Commission Staff Working Paper, *Assessment of the Implementation of the 2001 Employment Guidelines, Supporting Document to the Joint Employment Report 2001*. Brussels, 16.11.2001. Office for the Official

Publications of the European Communities, Luxembourg.

European Commission (2001d) The EU Economy 2001 Review. *European Economy* No. 73, 2001. www.europa.eu.int/comm/economy_finance/publications/european_economy/2001

European Commission (2002a) *Commission Recommendation for the 2002 Broad Guidelines of the Economic Policies of the Member States and the Community*. Brussels, 24.04.2002. www.europa.eu.int/comm/economy_finance/publications/europan_economy/2002/ee402en.pdf (accessed 23 March 2005).

European Commission (2002b) Commission Staff Working Paper. *Assessment of the Implementation of the 2002 Employment Guidelines. Supporting document to the Joint Employment Report 2002*. Brussels, 28.11.2002 SEC(2002) 1204/2. Office for the Official Publications of the European Communities, Luxembourg.

European Commission (2002c) *Communication from the Commission on Streamlining the Annual Economic and Employment Policy Coordination Cycles*. Brussels, 3.9.2002 COM(2002) 487 final. Office for the Official Publications of the European Communities, Luxembourg.

European Commission (2002d) Communication from the Commission to the Spring European Council in Barcelona. *The Lisbon Strategy – making change happen*. Brussels, 15.1.2002 COM(2002) 14 final. www.eu.eu.int/pressData/en/misc/69858.pdf (accessed 23 March 2005).

European Commission (2002e) Communication from the Commission to the Council and the European Parliament. *Strengthening the Coordination of Budgetary Policies*. Brussels, 27.11.2002 COM(2002) 668 final. www.europa.eu.int/eur-lex/en/com/cnc/2002/com2002_0668en01.pdf (accessed 2 March 2005).

European Commission (2003) Report on the implementation of the 2002 Broad Economic Policy Guidelines. *European Economy*. No. 1, January 2003. www.europa.eu.int/comm/economy_finance/publications/european_economy/2003/ec102en.pdf (accessed 23 March 2005).

European Court of Justice (1974) *Case 41/74*, van Duyn, ECR359.

European Parliament (1998) *Resolution on Democratic Accountability in the Third Phase of EM*. European Parliament, Brussels.

European Scrutiny Committee (2002) *The Committee's Work in 2002*. House of Commons, London.

Eve RA, Horsfall S and Lee ME (eds) (1997) *Chaos, Complexity and Sociology: myths, models and theories*. Sage, London.

EWCB (European Works Councils Bulletin) (May/June 1997) The Renault Vilvoorde affair. *EWCB*. **Issue 9**.

Falkner G (1998) *EU Social Policy in the 1990s: towards a corporatist policy community*. Routledge, London.

Farnham D and Pimlott J (1995) *Understanding Industrial Relations* (5e). Cassel, London.

Fatás A and Mihov I (2000) *Fiscal Policy and EMU: challenges of the early years. INSEAD and CEPR*. (www.faculty.insead.fr/mihov/files/FRemu(final).pdf (accessed 4 September 2004).

Featherstone K (1999) The political dynamics of Economic and Monetary Union. In: L Cram, D Dinan and N Nugent (eds) *Developments in the European Union*. Macmillan, Basingstoke. 311–29.

Ferrera M and Rhodes M (eds) (2000) Recasting European welfare states. Special issue of *West European Politics*. 23.

Fraser D (1973) *The Evolution of the British Welfare State*. Macmillan, London.

FT.com *Financial Times* (9 September 2001) Pedro Solbes tells Peter Norman he is a strong believer in the controversial mechanism to safeguard the euro. www.specials.ft.com/euro/FT39PUR31RC.html (accessed 7 April 2005).

FT.com *Financial Times* (1 February 2002) The real restraint on Germany. www.specials.ft.com/euro/FT36LRNC5XC.html (accessed 2 March 2005).

FT.com *Financial Times* (10 February 2002) EU faces showdown on warning to Germany. www.news.ft.com (accessed 2 March 2005).

FT.com *Financial Times* (14 February 2002) Editorial Comment: Europe's whipping boy. www.news.ft.com/ft/gx.cgi/ftc?pagename=View&c=Article&cid=FT34LF00PXC&live=true (accessed 7 April 2005).

FT.com *Financial Times* (20 May 2002) Euro's triumphant start leaves many challenges. www.specials.ft.com/euro/FT3RUEK8G1D.html (accessed 2 March 2005).

FT.com *Financial Times* (21 May 2002) Irish budget problems loom for government. www.specials.ft.com/euro/ (accessed 2 March 2005).

FT.com *Financial Times* (30 June 2003) Berlin tax plan tests EU rules on deficits. www.specials.ft.com (accessed 7 April 2005)

Fukuyama F (1993) *The End of History and the Last Man*. Penguin. London.

Fukuyama F (2001) How the West has won. *The Guardian*. 11 October.

Fuller S (1997) *Science*. Open University Press, Buckingham.

Gamble A (2001) *Europeanisation: a political economy perspective*. The Europeanisation of British Public and Social Policy, PAC/JUC Residential School, York.

Geddes A (1993) *Britain in the European Community*. Baseline Books, Manchester.

Gell-Mann M (1994) *The Quark and the Jaguar*. Little Brown, London.

George S (1991) *An Awkward Partner: Britain in the European Community*. Oxford University Press, Oxford.

Geyer R (1996) Globalisation and the (non-) defence of the welfare state. *West European Politics*. **21**: 77–102.

Geyer R (1997) *The Uncertain Union: British and Norwegian Social Democrats in an integrating Europe*. Avebury, Aldershot.

Geyer R (2000a) Can mainstreaming save EU Social Policy? The cases of gender, disability and elderly policy. *Current Politics and Economics of Europe*. **10**: 2.

Geyer R (2000b) *Exploring European Social Policy*. Polity Press, Cambridge.

Geyer R (2001) Can European Union Social NGOs co-operate to promote EU social policy? *Journal of Social Policy*. **30**: 3.

Geyer R (2003a) European integration, the problem of complexity and the revision of theory. *Journal of Common Market Studies*. **41**: 15–35.

Geyer R (2003b) Beyond the Third Way: the science of complexity and politics of choice. *British Journal of Politics and International Relations*. **5**: 237–57.

Geyer R (2003c) The end of globalisation and Europeanisation, rise of complexity and future of Scandinavian exceptionalism. *Governance*. 16: 4.

Geyer R and Rihani S (2001) Complexity: an appropriate framework for development? *Progress in Development Studies*. 1: 237–45.

Geyer R and Springer B (1998) EU social policy after Maastricht: the Works Council Directive and British opt-out. In: P Laurent and M Maresceau (eds) *The State of the European Union* Vol. 4. Lynne Rienner, Boulder, CO.

Giddens A (1994) *Beyond Left and Right: the future of radical politics.* Polity Press, Oxford.

Giddens A (1998) *The Third Way: the renewal of social democracy.* Polity Press, Cambridge.

Giddens A (2000) *The Third Way and its Critics.* Polity Press, Cambridge.

Giordano F and Persaud S (1998) *The Political Economy of Monetary Union. Towards the Euro.* Routledge, London.

Gladstone A (1993) Information and consultation in European multinationals: report on the Copenhagen Conference (April 1991). In: M Gold (ed.) *P+ European Participation Monitor.* Issue 6.

Gleick J (1988) *Chaos.* Sphere, London.

Glennerster H (2000) *British Social Policy Since 1945.* Blackwell Publishers, Oxford.

Goetschy J (2000) The European Employment Strategy: strength and weakness of an open method of coordination. Paper published by *ECSA (American political science journal)*, Wisconsin University, USA. **13**(3), Autumn 2000. www.ui.se/texter/janine.pdf (accessed 2 March 2005).

Goetschy J (2001) The European Employment Strategy from Amsterdam to Stockholm: has it reached its cruising speed? *Industrial Relations Journal.* **23**: 401–17.

Gold M (ed.) (1993) *The Social Dimension: employment policy in the European Community.* Macmillan, Basingstoke.

Goodin R, Headey B, Muffles R and Dirven H-J (1999) *The Real Worlds of Welfare Capitalism.* Cambridge University Press, Cambridge.

Goodman J, Marchington M, Berridge J, Snape E and Bamber GJ (1998) Employment relations in Britain. In: GJ Bamber and RD Lansbury (eds) *International Comparative Employment Relations. A study of industrialised market economies.* Sage Publications, London.

Gormley W (ed.) (1998) *Introduction to the Law of the European Communities from Maastricht to Amsterdam* (3e). Kluwer Law International, London.

Goss D and Adam-Smith D (2001) Pragmatism and compliance: employer responses to the Working Time Regulations. *Industrial Law Journal.* **32**: 195–208.

Gough I (1979) *The Political Economy of the Welfare State.* Macmillan, London.

Government Office for the North West – Structural Funds. www.go-nw.gov.uk (accessed 2 March 2005).

Gowland D and Turner A (2000) *Reluctant Europeans: Britain and European Integration 1945–1998.* Pearson Education Limited, Harlow.

Grebogi C and Yorke J (eds) (1997) *The Impact of Chaos on Science and Society.* United Nations University Press, Tokyo.

Gros D and Thygesen N (1998) *European Monetary Integration: from the European Monetary System to Economic and Monetary Union* (2e). Addison Wesley Longman, Harlow.

Guardian (13 February 2001) Brown sees off Brussels attack on spending.

Guardian (29 December 2001) The euro delusion.

Gulbenkian Commission (1996) *Open the Social Sciences.* Stanford University Press, Stanford.

Haas E (1970) The study of regional integration: the joys and anguish of pre-theorising. *International Organization.* **24**: 4.

Hall M (1992) Legislating for employee participation: a case study of the European Works Councils Directive. *Warwick Papers in Industrial Relations* No. 39, March.

Hall M (1994) Industrial relations and the social dimension of European integration: before and after Maastricht. In: R Hyman and A Ferner (eds) *New Frontiers in European Industrial Relations.* Blackwell Publishers, Oxford. 281–311.

Hall MM, Carley M, Gold P, Marginson P and Sisson K (1995) *European Works Councils - planning for the Directive.* Industrial Relations Research Unit, Warwick.

Hall S (1998) The Great Going Nowhere Show. *Marxism Today.* November/December, 9–14.

Hanson CG (1991) *Taming the Trade Unions: a guide to the Thatcher Government's Employment Reforms, 1980–1990.* Macmillan, Basingstoke.

Hantrais L (2002) *Social Policy in the European Union* (2e). Macmillan, Basingstoke.

Hatt S (1997) *Gender, Work and Labour Markets.* Macmillan Press Ltd, Basingstoke.

Hawking S (1988) *A Brief History of Time.* Bantam Books, New York.

Hay C (2001) Globalization, economic change and the welfare state: the vexatious inquisition of taxation. In: R Sykes, D Palier and P Prior (eds) *Globalization and European Welfare States: challenges and change.* Palgrave, London. 38–58.

Hay C (2002) *Political Analysis: a critical introduction.* Palgrave, London.

Hayek FA (1967) *Studies in Philosophy, Politics and Economics.* University of Chicago Press, Chicago.

Healey NM (2000) The case for European Monetary Union. In: M Baimbridge, B Burkitt and P Whyman (eds) *The Impact of the Euro. Debating Britain's Future.* Macmillan, Basingstoke.

Heath E (2000) Sovereignty in the modern world. In: M Baimbridge, B Burkitt and P Whyman (eds) *The Impact of the Euro. Debating Britain's Future.* Macmillan, Basingstoke.

Hepple B (1998) United Kingdom. In: European Commission (ed.) *The Regulation of Working Conditions in the Member States of the European Union, Volume 2. The legal systems of the Member States; a comparative perspective.* National Reports, Office for Official Publications of the European Communities, Luxembourg.

Hine D (1998) Introduction. The European Union, state autonomy and national social policy. In D Hine and H Kassim (eds) *Beyond the Market: the EU and national social policy.* Routledge, London.

Hine D and Kassim H (1998) *Beyond the Market: the EU and national social policy* Routledge, London.

Hirst P and Thompson G (1996) *Globalization in Question.* Polity Press, Cambridge.

HM Treasury (1999a) *Analysing UK Fiscal Policy.* www.hm-treasury.gov.uk/pdf/1999/anfiscalp.pdf (accessed 4 September 2004).

HM Treasury (1999b) *The New Monetary Policy Framework.* www.hm-treasury.gov.uk/pdf/1999/monetary.pdf (accessed 23 March 2005).

HM Treasury (2000) *Delivering Economic Stability. Convergence Programme Submitted in line with the Stability and Growth Pact. December 2000.* www.hm-treasury.gov.uk/pdf/2000/convergence221200.pdf (accessed 23 March 2005).

HM Treasury (2001) *UK Policy Coordination: the importance of institutional design.* www.hm-treasury.gov.uk/docs/2001/institutional_design.html

HM Treasury (2002a) *Realising Europe's Potential: economic reform in Europe.* www.hm-treasury.gov.uk/mediastore/otherfiles/eer_wp02chaps1to2.pdf (accessed 23 March 2005).

HM Treasury (2002b) *Sustainability for the Long Term: convergence programme for the United Kingdom, Submitted in line with the Stability and Growth Pact, December 2002.* www.hm-treasury.gov.uk/media//8F989/convergprogfinal02.pdf (accessed 2 March 2005).

HM Treasury, DTI and DWP (2002) *Towards Full Employment in the European Union, July 2002.* www.hmtreasury.gov.uk/mediastore/otherfiles/towards_full_employment+1.pdf (accessed 23 March 2005).

Hodgson G (1997) *Economics and Evolution.* University of Michigan Press, Ann Arbor.

Hodson D and Maher I (2001) The open method as a new mode of governance. *Journal of Common Market Studies.* **39**: 719–46.

Hooghe L and Marks G (2001) *Multi-level Governance and European Integration.* Rowman and Littlefield, Lanham.

Horgan J (1996) *The End of Science.* Addison-Wesley, Reading, MA.

Hoskyns C (1996) *Integrating Gender: women, law and politics in the European Union.* Verso, London.

House of Commons (1998) www.parliament.uk

Independent (23 October 2002) Analysis: 'Stupidity pact' crumbles as euro's foundation stone. www.news.independent.co.uk/europe/story/jsp?story=345044 (accessed 7 April 2005).

Jackman R (1998) The impact of the European Union on unemployment and unemployment policy. In: D Hine and K Kassim (eds) *Beyond the Market: the EU and national social policy.* Routledge, London. 60–78.

Jervis R (1997) *System Effects.* Princeton University Press, Princeton, NJ.

Johnson C (1996) *In With the Euro, Out With the Pound: the single currency for Britain.* Penguin Books, London.

Jones B (1994) Conservatism. In: B Jones, A Gray, D Kavanagh *et al.* (eds) *Politics UK* (2e). Harvester Wheatsheaf, Hemel Hempstead. 125–39.

Jørgensen KE (ed.) (1997) *Reflective Approaches to European Governance.* Macmillan, Basingstoke.

Katzenstein P, Keohane R and Krasner S (1998) International organization and the study of world politics. *International Organization.* **52**: 645–85.

Kauffman S (1993) *The Origins of Order.* Oxford University Press, Oxford.

Kauffman S (1995) *At Home in the Universe.* Viking, London.

Kenner J (1999) The EC employment title and the 'Third Way': making soft law work. *International Journal of Comparative Labour Law and Industrial Relations.* **15**: 33–60.

Keohane R and Nye J (1977) *Power and Interdependence: world politics in transition.* Little Brown, Boston.

Kiel LD and Elliot E (eds) (1997) *Chaos Theory in the Social Sciences: foundation and application.* University of Michigan Press, Ann Arbor.

King A (ed.) (1976) *Why is Britain Becoming Harder to Govern?* BBC, London.

Kleinman M (2002) *A European Welfare State? European Union social policy in context*. Palgrave, Basingstoke.

Knill C (2001) *The Europeanisation of National Administration*. Cambridge University Press, Cambridge.

Krasner S (1983*) International Regimes*. Cornell University Press, Ithaca.

Krasner S (ed.) (1990) *The Ubiquity of Chaos*. The American Association for the Advancement of Science, Washington DC.

Krieger J (1986) *Reagan, Thatcher and the Politics of Decline*. Oxford University Press, Oxford.

Kuhn T (1970) *The Structure of Scientific Revolutions*. University of Chicago Press, Chicago.

Kuhnle S (2000) *Survival of the European Welfare State*. Routledge, London.

Labour Party (1983) *General Election Manifesto.* Labour Party, London.

Labour Party (1997a) *Britain will be better with New Labour.* www.labourwin97.org.uk (accessed September 2004).

Labour Party (1997b) *Equipping Britain for the Future*. Labour Party, London.

Lafointaine O (1998) The future of German Social Democracy. *New Left Review.* **227**: 72–87.

Larsson A (1999*) The European Employment Strategy: towards the Helsinki Summit – 'putting Europe to work'. Eskilstuna*, 9 December 1999 (speech).

Lawzone (6 September 2000) *Is 'On-Call' Time Working Time?* www.lawzone.co.uk/cgi-bin/item.cgi?id=25844&d-pndp&h-pnhp&f-pnfp (accessed 2 March 2005).

Lawzone (2002a, 10 February) *Territorial Reach of the Working Time Regulations*. www.lawzone.co.uk/cgi-bin/item.cgi?id=71651 (accessed 2 March 2005).

Lawzone (2002b, 30 May) *New EAT Decision.* www.lawzone.co.uk/cgi-bin/item.cgi?id=82291 (accessed 2 March 2005).

Layard R (2000) Joining Europe's currency. In: M Baimbridge, B Burkitt and P Whyman (eds) *The Impact of the Euro: debating Britain's future*. Macmillan, Basingstoke.

Leibfried S and Obinger H (eds) (2000) *Focus: the future of the welfare state*. Special issue of *European Review: Interdisciplinary Journal of the Academia Europaea*. **8**: 3.

Leibfried S and Pierson P (eds) (1995) *European Social Policy: between fragmentation and integration*. The Brookings Institute, Washington DC.

Leibfried S and Pierson P (1996) In: W Wallace and H Wallace (eds) *Policy Making in the European Union*. Oxford University Press, Oxford.

Levitt M and Lord C (2000) *The Political Economy of Monetary Union*. Macmillan, Basingstoke.

Levy J (1999) Vice into virtue? Progressive politics and welfare reform in continental Europe. *Politics and Society.* **27**: 239–73.

Lewin R (1999) *Complexity: life on the edge of chaos*. Prentice Hall, New York.

Liberal Democrat website. www.libdems.org.uk

Lightfoot S (1999) Prospects for Euro-socialism. *Renewal.* **7**: 7–17.

Lönnroth J (2002) Gender mainstreaming policy under the European Employment Strategy and the Social Inclusion Strategy. Conference on Gender Equality, Athens, 28 February 2002.

Lourie J (1998) *Working Time Regulations. House of Commons Library Research Paper 98/82*, 10 August 1998. www.parliament.uk/commons/lib/research/

rp98/rp98–082.pdf (accessed September 2004).

Lovelock J (1979) *Gaia: a new look at life on Earth*. Oxford University Press, Oxford.

Lyotard J-F (1993) *The Postmodern Condition: a report on knowledge*. University of Minnesota Press, Minneapolis.

MacDougall D (Sir) (2001) Unwillingness to help each other adds to euro risk. Letters to the Editor, *Financial Times*, 16 February 2001.

Mainzer K (1997) *Thinking in Complexity: the computational dynamics of matter, mind and mankind* (3e). Springer, Berlin.

Marginson P and Sisson K (1994) The structure of transnational capital in Europe: the emerging Euro-company and its implications for industrial relations. In: R Hyman and A Ferner (eds) *New Frontiers in European Industrial Relations*. Blackwell, Oxford. 15–51.

Marginson P and Sisson K (2001) *European Dimensions to Collective Bargaining: new symmetries within an asymmetric process?* Paper for the 6th European IIRA Congress, Oslo, 25–29 June 2001. www.users.wbs.warwick.ac.uk/irru/publications/conference_papers/012marginson.pdf (accessed 2 March 2005).

Marks G *et al.* (1996) European integration from the 1980s: State-centric v. multi-level governance. *Journal of Common Market Studies*. **34**: 341–78.

Marks G and McAdam D (1996) Social movements and the changing structure of political opportunity in the European Union. In: G Marks, F Scharpf, P Schmitter and W Streeck (eds) *Governance in the European Union*. Sage, London.

Marshall T (1964) *Class, Citizenship and Social Development*. Doubleday, Garden City, NY.

Martin D (1989) A Left agenda for Europe. *Contemporary European Affairs*. **1**(1): 109–29.

Martin M and McIntyre L (1994) *Readings in the Philosophy of Social Science*. MIT Press, Cambridge, MA.

Mattli W and Slaughter A (1995) Law and politics in the European Union: a reply to Garrett. *International Organization*. **49**: 1.

Mazey S (1998) The European Union and women's rights: from Europeanisation of national agendas to the nationalisation of a European agenda. In: D Hine and H Kassim (eds) *Beyond the Market. The EU and national social policy*. Routledge, London. 134–56.

Mazey S (2001) *Gender Mainstreaming in the EU: Principles and Practice*. Kogan Page Limited, London.

McColgan A (2000a) Family friendly frolics? The Maternity and Parental Leave etc. Regulations 1999. *Industrial Law Journal*. **29**(2): 125–44.

McColgan A (2000b) Missing the point? The Part-time Workers (Prevention of Less Favourable Treatment) Regulations 2000 (SI 2000, No. 1551). *Industrial Law Journal*. **29**(3): 260–6.

McKay S (2001) Annual Review Article 2000. Between flexibility and regulation: rights, equality and protection at work. *British Journal of Industrial Relations*. **39**: 285–303.

Meulders D and Plasman R (1997) European economic policies and social quality. In: W Beck, L van der Maesen and A Walker (eds) *The Social Quality of Europe*. Kluwer, The Hague. 19–41.

Miliband R (1973) *The State in Capitalist Society*. Quartet Books, London.

Millward NA, Bryson A and Forth J (1998) *All Change At Work? British employment relations 1980–1998, as portrayed by the Workplace Industrial Relations Survey series*. Routledge, London.

Minford P (2000) The Single Currency – will it work and should we join? In: M Baimbridge, B Burkitt and P Whyman (eds) *The Impact of the Euro: debating Britain's future*. Macmillan, Basingstoke.

Mirowski P (1994) *Natural Images in Economic Thought*. Cambridge University Press, Cambridge.

Moffat G (1998) *The Regulation of Working Time: a European Odyssey*. Warwick Papers in Industrial Relations, Number 60. Industrial Relations Research Unit, University of Warwick, Coventry.

Moran M (1994) The social and economic structure. In: B Jones, A Gray, D Kavanagh *et al.* (eds) *Politics UK* (2e). Harvester Wheatsheaf, Hemel Hempstead. 63–93.

Moravcsik A (1993) Preference and power in the European Community: a liberal intergovernmental approach. *Journal of Common Market Studies*. **31**: 473–524.

Moravcsik A (2001) Constructivism and European integration: a critique. In: T Christiansen, K Jørgensen and A Wiener (eds) *The Social Construction of Europe*. Sage, London. 176–89.

Morgenthau H (1960) *Politics Among Nations: the struggle for power and peace* (3e). Knopf, New York.

Moses J (1994) Abdication from national policy autonomy: what's left to leave. *Politics and Society*. **22**: 125–48.

Müller T and Hoffmann A (2001) *EWC Research: a review of the literature*. Warwick Papers in Industrial Relations, No. 65, November. Industrial Relations Research Unit. www.users.wbs.warwick.ac.uk/irru/publications/paper_65.pdf (accessed 2 March 2005).

Neathy F and Arrowsmith J (2001) *Implementation of the Working Time Regulations*. Department of Trade and Industry, Employment Relations Research Series No. 11. www.dti.gov.uk/er/emor/wtr.pdf (accessed September 2004).

Newman J (2000) Beyond the new public management? Modernizing public services. In: J Clarke, S Gewirtz and E McLaughlin (eds) *New Managerialism, New Welfare?* Sage, London. 45–62.

Nicolis G and Prigogine I (1989) *Exploring Complexity*. Freeman, New York.

Nott S (1999) Mainstreaming equal opportunities: succeeding when all else has failed. In: A Morris and T O'Donnell (eds) *Feminist Perspectives on Employment Law*. Cavendish Publishing Limited, London.

Ohmae K (1990) *The Borderless World*. HarperCollins, New York.

Ohmae K (1995) *The End of the Nation-State*. Jossey Bass Wiley, New York.

Onuf N (1989) *A World of Our Making: rules and rule in social theory and international relations*. University of South Carolina Press, Columbia.

Ormerod P (1994) *The Death of Economics*. Faber and Faber, London.

Ormerod P (1998) *Butterfly Economics*. Faber and Faber, London.

Pierson C (1999) *Beyond the Welfare State? The new political economy of welfare*. Polity Press, Oxford.

Pilkington C (2001) *Britain in the European Union Today*. Manchester University Press, Manchester.

Pochet P (1999) The New Employment Chapter of the Amsterdam Treaty.

Journal of European Social Policy. **9**: 271–8.

Pollack M (2001) International relations theory and European integration. *Journal of Common Market Studies.* **39**: 221–44.

Powell M (ed.) (1999) *New Labour, New Welfare State? The Third Way in British Social Policy.* The Policy Press, Bristol.

Prakash A and Hart J (1999) *Globalization and Governance.* Routledge, London.

Puchala D (1972) Of blind men, elephants and international integration. *Journal of Common Market Studies.* **10**: 3.

Radaelli C (2001) *The Europeanisation of Public Policy: notes on theory, methods and the challenge of empirical research.* Department of Public Policy, Bradford University, Bradford. www.york.ac.uk/depts/poli/juc/2001/crpaper.htm

Rasch W and Wolfe C (eds) (2000) *Observing Complexity: systems theory and post-modernity.* University of Minnesota Press, Minneapolis.

Redwood J (2000) In: M Baimbridge, B Burkitt and P Whyman (eds) *The Impact of the Euro: debating Britain's future.* Macmillan, Basingstoke.

Rees T (1998) *Mainstreaming Equality in the European Union: education, training and labour market policies.* Routledge, London.

Rees T (2002) *Gender Mainstreaming: misappropriated and misunderstood?* Paper presented to the Department of Sociology, University of Sweden, 21 February 2002. www.sociology.su.se/cgs/ReesPaper.doc (accessed 2 March 2005).

Rengger N (2000) *International Relations, Political Theory and the Problem of Order.* Routledge, London.

Rhodes M (1996) Globalization, labour markets and welfare states: a future of competitive corporatism. *Journal of European Social Policy.* **6**: 305–27.

Rhodes M and Meny Y (1998) *The Future of European Welfare: a new social contract?* Macmillan, London.

Richards D and Smith MJ (2002) *Governance and Public Policy in the UK.* Oxford University Press, Oxford.

Richardson K and Cilliers P (2001) What is Complexity Science? A view from different directions. *Emergence.* **3**: 5–22.

Rihani S (2002) *Complex Systems Theory and Development Practice: understanding non-linear realities.* Zed Books, London.

Rihani S and Geyer R (2001) Complexity: a new framework for development theory. *Progress in Development Studies.* **1**(3).

Roelofs E (1995) The European Equal Opportunities Policy. In: A van Doorne-Huiskes, J van Hoof and E Roelofs (eds) *Women and the European Labour Markets.* Open University, Heerlen, The Netherlands.

Room G (1994) European social policy: competition, conflict and integration. In: R Page and J Baldock (eds) *Social Policy Review 6.* Social Policy Association, Canterbury. 17–35.

Rosamond B (2000) *Theories of European Integration.* Macmillan, London.

Rose N (1999) Inventiveness in politics. *Economy and Society.* **28**: 467–93.

Rose R (1993) *Lesson Drawing in Public Policy.* Chatham House, Chatham, NJ.

Rouse J and Smith G (1999) Accountability. In: M Powell (ed.) *New Labour, New Welfare State? The 'Third Way' in British social policy.* The Policy Press, Bristol. 235–56.

Ruggie J (1982) International regimes, transactions, and change: embedded liberalism in the postwar economic order. *International Organization.* **36**: 2.

Ryan A (1999) Britain: recycling the Third Way. *Dissent.* **46**: 77–80.

Rycroft R and Kash D (1999) *The Complexity Challenge: technological innovation for the 21st century*. Pinter, London.

Sandholtz W (1996) Membership matters: limits of the functional approach to European institutions. *Journal of Common Market Studies*. **34**: 3.

Sarfati H (1998) Negotiating trade-offs between jobs and labour market flexibility in the European Union. *International Journal of Comparative Labour Law and Industrial Relations*. **14**: 307–24.

Scharpf F (1991) *Crisis and Choice in European Social Democracy*. Cornell University Press, Ithaca.

Schmitter P (1996) Some alternative futures for the European policy and their implications for European public policy. In: Y Yves Meny, P Muller and J–L Quermonne (eds) *Adjusting to Europe: the impact of the European Union on national institutions and policies*. Routledge, London. 25–40.

Sciarra S (1999) The employment title in the Amsterdam Treaty: a multi-language legal discourse. In: D O'Keefe and P Twomey (eds) *Legal Issues of the Amsterdam Treaty*. Hart Publishing, Oxford. 157–70.

Scott J (1998) *Seeing Like a State*. Yale University Press, New Haven.

Shonefield A (1972) *Europe: journey to an unknown destination*. Penguin Books, London.

Smith DH (1973) *Confucius*. Temple Smith, London.

Smith E (1998) *Will EMU Lead to Political Union?* Centre for European Reform Online (October 1998). www.cer.org.uk/articles/n_2_4.html (accessed 2 March 2005).

Smith S (2001a) Reflectivist and constructivist approaches to international theory. In: J Baylis and S Smith (eds) *The Globalization of World Politics: an introduction to international relations* (2e). Oxford University Press, Oxford. 271–96.

Smith S (2001b) Social constructivisms and European studies. In: T Christiansen, K Jørgensen and A Wiener (eds) *The Social Construction of Europe*. Sage, London. 189–99.

Sole R and Goodwin B (2001) *Signs of Life: how complexity pervades biology*. Basic Books, New York.

Squires J and Wickham-Jones M (2002) Mainstreaming in Westminster and Whitehall: from Labour's Ministry for Women to the Women and Equality Unit. *Parliamentary Affairs*: *A Journal of Comparative Politics*. **55**: 57–70.

Stacey R (1999) *Strategic Management and Organisational Dynamics: the challenge of complexity* (3e). Financial Times/Prentice Hall, London.

Stacey R, Griffin D and Shaw P (2000) *Complexity and Management: fad or radical challenge to systems thinking?* Routledge, London.

Stewart M (1984) *The Age of Interdependence: economic policy in a shrinking world*. MIT Press, Cambridge, MA.

Stone D (1999) Learning lessons and transferring policy across time, space and disciplines. *Politics*. **19**: 51–9.

Streeck W (1996) Neo-Voluntarism: a new European Social Policy regime. In: G Marks, F Scharpf, P Schmitter and W Streeck (eds) *Governance in the European Union*. Sage, London. 64–95.

Streeck W (1998) The internationalisation of industrial relations in Europe: prospects and problems. *Politics and Society*. **26**: 429–59.

Strong H (1962) *Essays on the Scientific Study of Politics*. Holt, Rinehart and Winston, New York.

Sunday Times (18 February 2001) Brown launches a phoney war to hide his euro hand.

Swank D (1998) Funding the welfare state: globalisation and the taxation of business in advanced market economies. *Political Studies.* **46**: 671–92.

Sykes R and Alcock P (eds) (1998) *Developments in European Social Policy: convergence and diversity.* The Policy Press, Bristol.

Sykes R, Palier B and Prior P (eds) (2001) *Globalization and European Welfare States: challenges and change.* Palgrave, London.

Szyszczak E (2000a) *EC Labour Law.* Pearson Education Limited, Harlow.

Szyszczak E (2000b) The evolving European Employment Strategy. In: J Shaw (ed.) *Social Law and Policy in an Evolving Europe.* Hart, Oxford. 197–222.

Taylor P (1983) *The Limits of European Integration.* Croom Helm, London.

Teeple G (1995) *Globalisation and the Decline of Social Reform.* Garamond, Toronto.

Temperton P (2001) *The UK and the Euro.* John Wiley and Sons Ltd, Chichester.

Thrift N (1999) The place of complexity. *Theory, Culture and Society.* **16** (3): 31–69.

The Times (29 May 2001) Jospin sets out vision of a more French EU. www.timesonline.co.uk (accessed 7 April 2005).

The Times (12 February 2001) Brown says euro will damage Britain.

Tondl G (2000) Fiscal federalism and the reality of the European Union Budget. In: C Crouch (ed.) *After The Euro: shaping institutions for governance in the wake of European Monetary Union.* Oxford University Press, Oxford. 227–56.

Tranholm-Mikkelsen J (1991) Neo-Functionalism: obstinate or obsolete. *Millennium.* **20**: 1–22.

Trubek DM and Mosher J (2001a) *New Governance, EU Employment Policy, and the European Social Model.* Symposium: Responses to the European Commission's White Paper on Governance. www.jeanmonnetprogram.org/papers/01/011501.html (accessed 2 March 2005).

Trubek DM and Mosher J (2001b) *New Governance, EU Employment Policy, and the European Social Model.* Paper presented at the Conference on Reconfiguring Work and Welfare in the New Economy, University of Wisconsin-Madison, 10–12 May.

Tsoukalis L (1993) *The New European Economy: the politics and economics of integration.* Oxford University Press, Oxford.

TUC (1998) *General Council Report 1998.* TUC, London.

TUC (2002) *One in six UK workers put in more than 48 hours a week.* Press Release, 4 February 2002. www.tuc.org.uk/work_life/tuc-4277-f0.cfm (accessed 2 March 2005).

Tucker C (2000) The Luxembourg Process: the UK view. *International Journal of Comparative Labour Law and Industrial Relations.* **16**: 71–83.

Undy R (1999) Annual Review Article: New Labour's Industrial Relations Settlement: The Third Way? *British Journal of Industrial Relations.* **37**: 315–36.

Waldrop M (1992) *Complexity: the emerging science at the edge of order and chaos.* Simon and Schuster, New York.

Waldrop M (1994) *Complexity: the emerging science at the edge of order and chaos.* Penguin Books Ltd, New York.

Walker RBJ (1993) *Inside/Outside: international relations as political theory.* Cambridge University Press, Cambridge.

Walsh K (1995) *Public Services and Market Mechanisms: competition, contracting and the new public management.* Macmillan, London.

Waltz K (1979) *Theory of International Politics.* McGraw-Hill, New York.

Weiler JHH (1991) The transformation of Europe. *Yale Law Journal.* **100**: 2403–83.

Wendt A (1992) Anarchy is what states make of it: the social construction of power politics. *International Organization.* **46**: 391–407.

Wendt A (1999) *Social Theory of International Politics.* Cambridge University Press, Cambridge.

Wilson EO (1999) *Consilience.* Random House, New York.

Wise M and Gibb R (1993) *Single Market to Social Europe.* Longman, Harlow.

Women and Equality Unit (WEU) (2003) *Delivering on Gender Equality: supporting the PSA objective on gender equality 2003–2006.* www.womenandequalityunit.gov.uk/research/delivering_on_gender.pdf (accessed 23 March 2005).

Index

Page numbers in *italics* refer to figures or tables.

Irish economy 151–2
Jenkins v. *Kingsgate (Clothing Productions Ltd)* (1981) 99
JERs *see* Joint Employment Reports
Joint Employment Reports (JERs) 83
  UK recommendations 83–4, 85, 87, 89

Kant, Immanuel 43–4
Katzenstein, P *et al.* 21
Kauffman, S 39
Kennedy, President John F 51
Kenner, J 78
Knill, Christoph 24
Kuhnle, Stein 10

Labour Government *see* New Labour
labour relations *see* EU labour relations policies; UK labour relations
Lafontaine, Oskar 156
Learndirect 82
legislation
  background history 7
  court rulings 10–11
  forms 7–8
  gender and equal opportunities 96–100
  and sovereignty 11
  UK Scrutiny Committee 11–12
Leigh-Pemberton, Robin 143
Leviathan (Hobbes) 41
Liberal Democrats, on EU social policy integration 14
Lifelong Learning Strategy 82
  and trade union/CBI involvement 85–7
'limited globalisation' 22
linearity principles 36, 41–2
  and European Union systems 59, 59
  and human complexity 48–9
  see also paradigm of order
Lisbon Summit (2000) 76–8, 156
litigation
  equal opportunities infringement proceedings 96–100
  labour relations infringements 123, 125, 131–2
Local Government International Bureau 15
Lorenzian Waterwheel 37
Lovelock, James 39–40
luck, and complexity theory 50
Luxembourg Process 4–5, 74–6
  and equal opportunities 110
  four pillars of employment reforms 75
Lyotard, Jean-Francois 44

Maastricht Treaty (1991/1993) 3–4, 13
  economic and monetary reform 142, 143
  and employment reform 72

McCreevy, Charlie 151–2
MacDougall Report (1977) 155
'mainstreaming' 5–6
  gender initiatives vs. disability/ageing initiatives 114–15
  and policy transfer (PT) theory 30–1
Mainzer, Klaus 54
Major, John 13, 143
Marshall v. *Southampton and South West Hants Area Health Authority* (1986) 99
Marxism 26–7
Marx, Karl 41
Maternity Allowance (MA) 104–5
maternity leave 86, 104–5
Mazey, S 94, 100
mechanistic complexity 49
methodological pluralism
  complexity theory 52–3, 53
  in EU and international systems 60–1
Michelson, Albert 33
migration policies *see* free movement policies
minimum wage *see* National Minimum Wage
Minister for Europe (UK) 9–10
MLG theory *see* multilevel governance (MLG) theory
modernist social science *see* orderly (modernist) social science
Monetary Policy committee (MPC) 143
Moravcsik, Andrew 22–3
Morgenthau, H 20
multilevel governance (MLG) theory 31

National Council for Voluntary Organisations 15
National Minimum Wage 103, 138
naturalists/anti-naturalists 52, 57
Neathey, F and Arrowsmith, J 133
neo-functionalism 22–3
New Deal initiatives 81–3
New Labour 4, 12–15, 162
  audit and control culture 63–4
  and EU equal opportunity policies 103–8, 111–12
  and EU labour relations policies 86, 123–4, 131–5, 137–9, 139
  family-friendly agenda 103–8
  and 'third way' (Giddens) 29, 63
New Liberalism 28
New Opportunities for Women (NOW) 109
Newtonian paradigm 33
  and complexity 53–5
  see also paradigm of order
Newton, Sir Isaac 33, 35